'HOW TO'

BOOK OF FIRST AID AND SAFETY

MARGARET NISBET

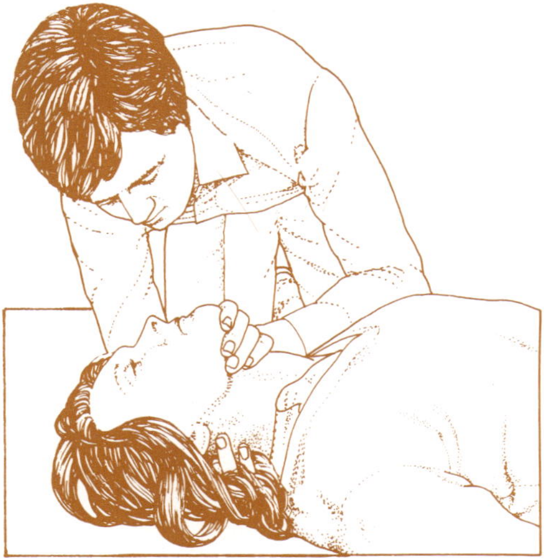

BROCKHAMPTON PRESS

'HOW TO'

The 'How To' Book of First Aid and Safety has been designed to make simple the techniques and methods which are essential in dealing effectively with accidents and emergencies in any situation.

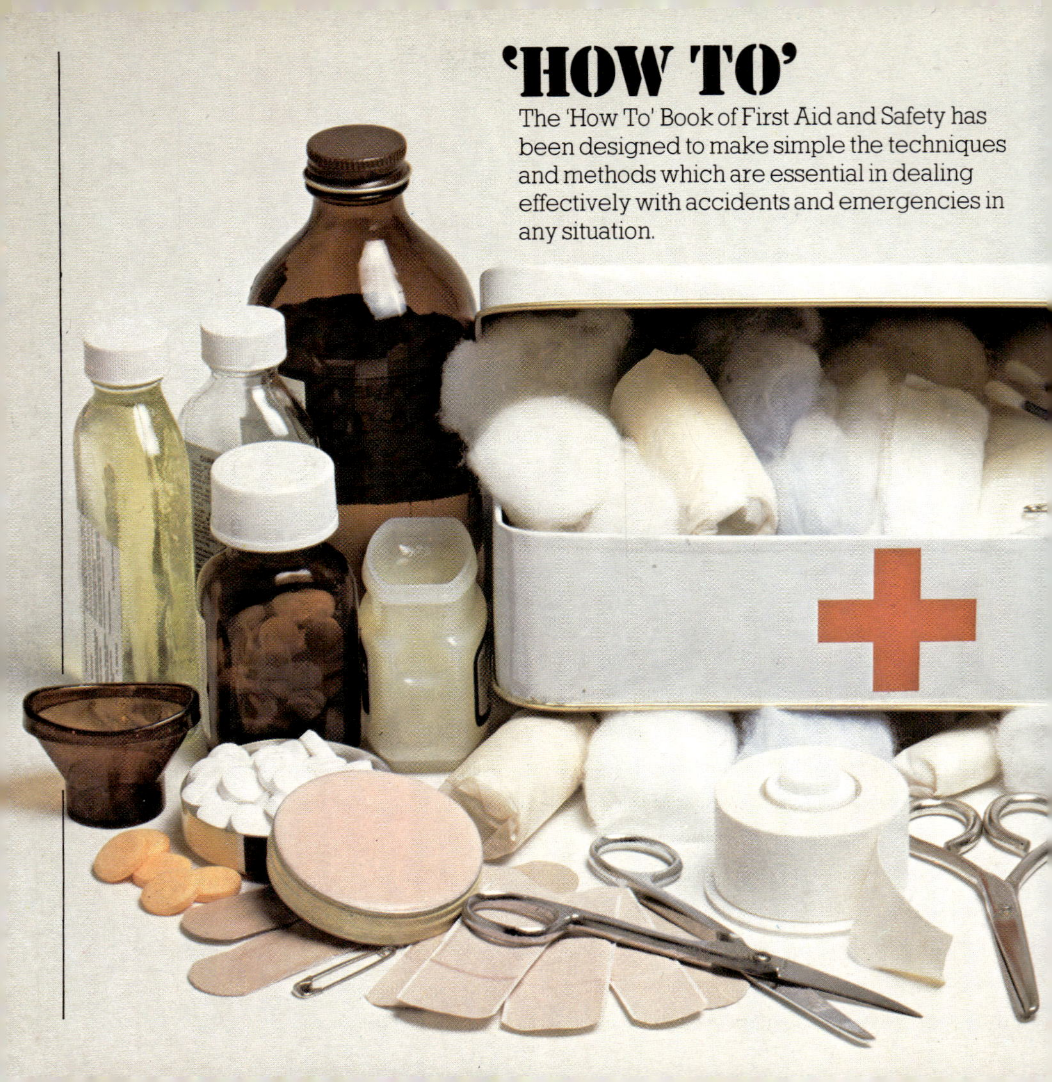

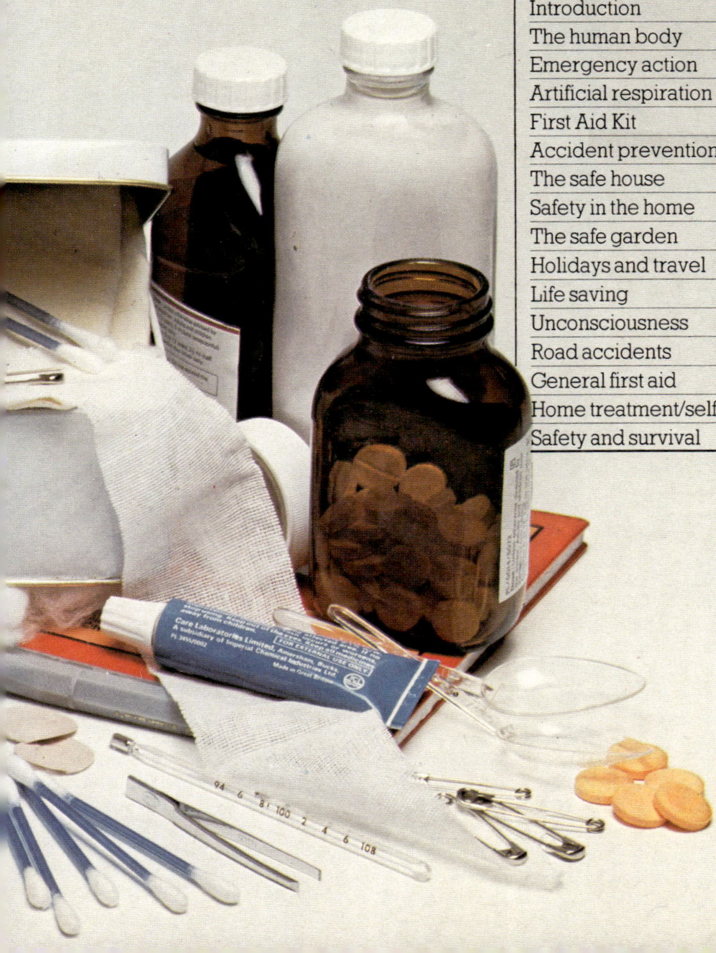

Contents

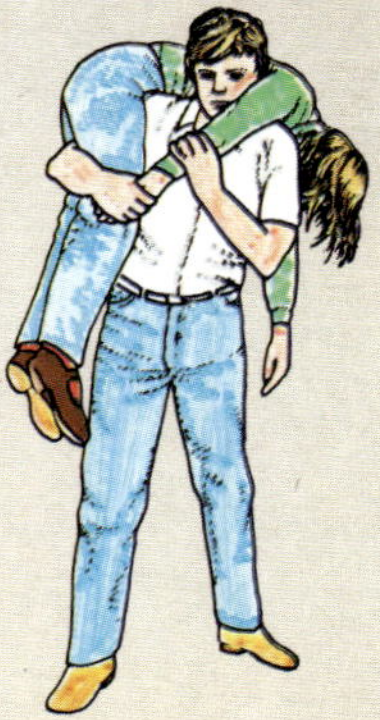

The 'How To' Book of First Aid and Safety was conceived, edited and designed by Simon Jennings and Company Limited, 42 Maiden Lane, London WC2, England

This edition published 1996 by Brockhampton Press Ltd, 20 Bloomsbury Street, London WC1B 3QA

ISBN 1 86019 234 3

Printed and bound in U.A.E.

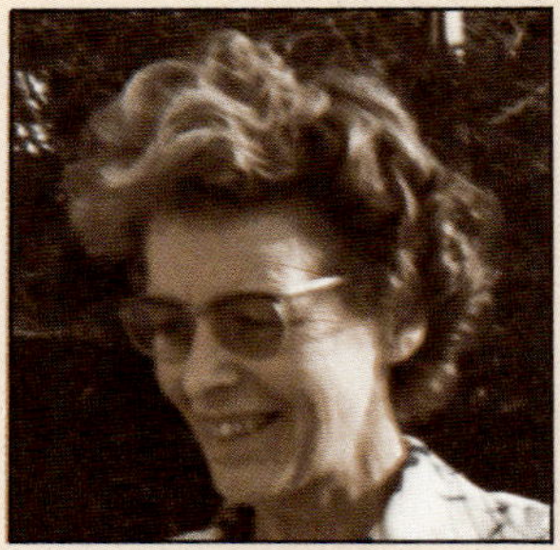

THE AUTHOR

Margaret Nisbet trained in orthopaedic and general nursing, then spent several years working for a prominent Forensic Pathologist in London. She subsequently joined the World Health Organisation in Geneva and later worked in Uganda, Denmark, India and Manila. After completing a course in journalism, she returned to the UN in Geneva and worked with a number of international agencies, including the International Council for Nurses. Margaret Nisbet now lives, with her journalist husband, in Dorset

Introduction

First Aid is the first help and treatment given to a person following injury or the onset of illness and is given before qualified medical assistance can be reached.

Modern life at home or elsewhere has a high accident risk. Few of us are able to take a detailed course to become qualified First Aid workers, but all of us – at some time – are likely to be first on the scene in an emergency. Knowing what to do first, and why, will give you confidence to carry out the essential treatment which may well save a life.

First Aid treatment has been very much simplified in recent years. There is no need to use complicated medical terms, but knowing a little of how the human body works will help you to understand the treatment and to recognise the implications of certain injuries.

The first and most important aims are to keep the injured person alive, to relieve suffering and prevent further injury, and to hand her over without delay for further treatment.

When you arrive on the scene of an accident: **1**. Find out what happened. **2**. Remove the victim from danger or danger from the victim (a badly injured person should not be moved except from continuing danger). Do not take unnecessary risks – you may become the next victim. **3**. Give essential treatment remembering the three priorities: ABC – Airways, Breathing, Circulation. Is the airway clear? Is she breathing? Is she bleeding? **4**. Send a message for a doctor or ambulance. **5**. Do not spend time on minor injuries. **6**. If the victim is conscious, reassure him and tell him what is happening.

Our charts and illustrations will help you to memorise these rules so that you can practise the procedures, know what a First Aid kit should contain, recognise common injuries and conditions, and treat minor ailments at home.

Many accidents can be prevented by making one's home as safe as possible. Emergencies will happen – but if you know your First Aid, you will be prepared to deal with them.

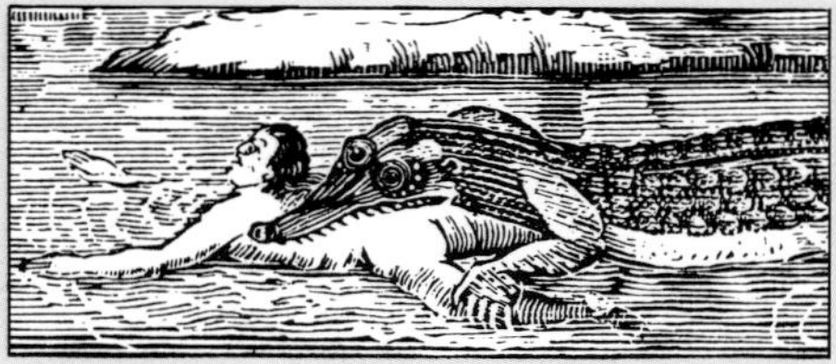

The human body

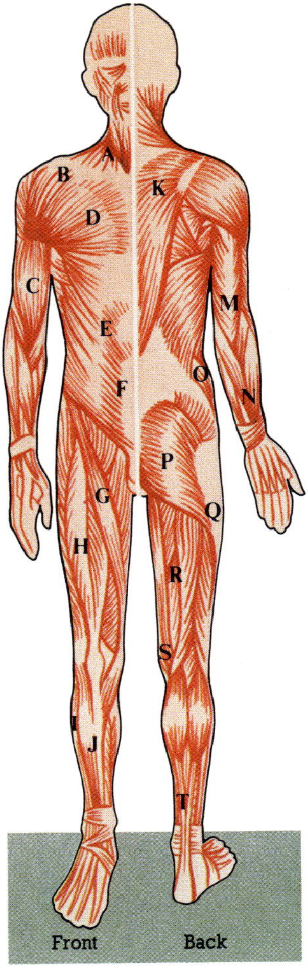

Basic muscles◄
Moving the human frame is a complex business. That is why we are equipped with 215 pairs of muscles to do the job. Those shown here are some of the most important.

● **Front**

- **A** Sternomastoid
- **B** Deltoid
- **C** Biceps
- **D** Pectoralis
- **E** External oblique
- **F** Rectus abdominus
- **G** Sartorius
- **H** Quadriceps
- **I** Peronei
- **J** Anterior tibial

● **Back**

- **K** Trapezius
- **M** Triceps
- **N** Flexors and extensors
- **O** External oblique
- **P** Gluteus maximus
- **Q** Tensor fasciae latae
- **R** Hamstrings
- **S** Sartorius
- **T** Soleus

The outer covering of the body is the skin, which protects the many interior tissues (made up of millions of cells) from injury and infection. The body is built on to a framework of muscles and bones which not only determine the body's shape, but also form a mechanical structure enabling it to move.

Where two or more bones meet, they form a joint. Some joints are fixed, while others have varying degrees of movement, such as ball-and-socket (hip) or hinge joints (elbow). To prevent friction, the rubbing surfaces of bones in movable joints are covered with smooth *cartilage*, and the joint is enclosed in a strong capsule which is strengthened by *ligaments*. This capsule is lined with a thin membrane, producing a fluid which 'oils' the joint.

Muscles are bundles of elastic fibres which are attached to the bones by *tendons*. They are called voluntary muscles, and their function is to produce movement in response to messages from the brain. They do this by working in pairs – one relaxing while the other contracts. Involuntary muscles work continuously in the internal organs, helping to maintain the smooth operating of the functions of the body.

The skeleton ▶
The most important bones of the body are shown on this page. These, in conjunction with the muscles, form the basis of the mechanical framework which enables the body to move.

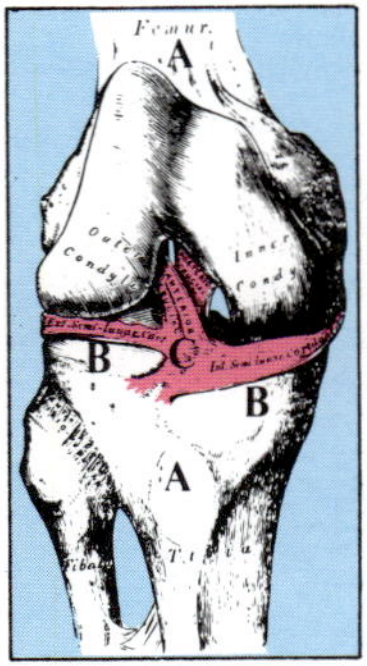

How a joint works
Movement is effected by muscles pulling against the bones. A joint is an arrangement of bone **(A),** cartilage **(B),** and ligament **(C):** ligaments to link the bones flexibly; cartilage to provide a protective cushion between the bones.

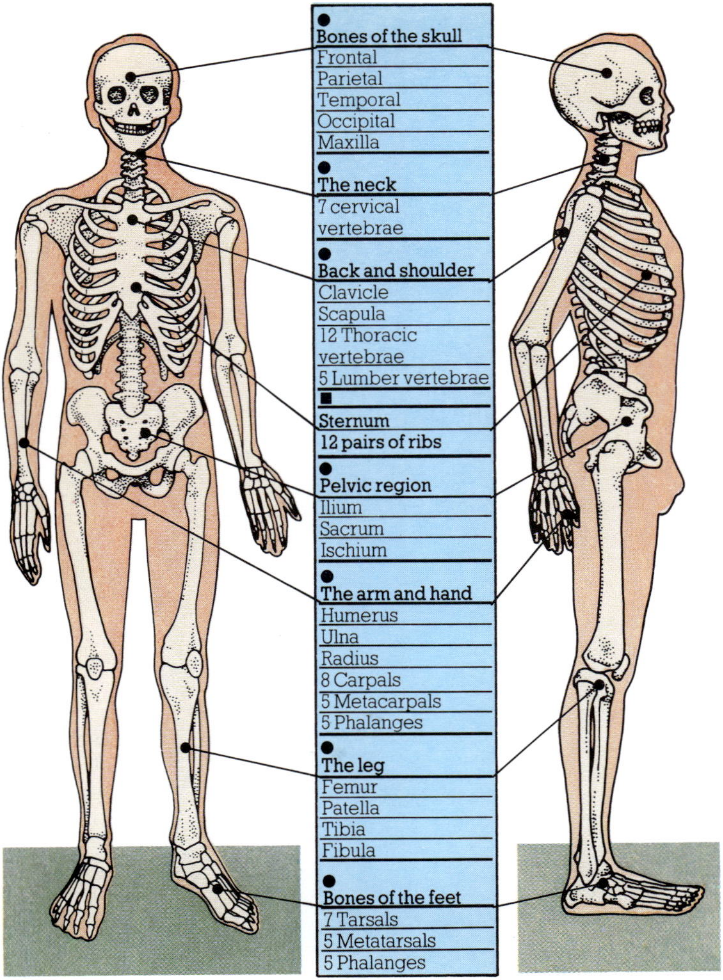

Emergency action

Is victim breathing?

Feel with your hand for any movement of chest or abdominal walls. Place your ear near his face – can you hear air being drawn in or blown out? If no movement of air into the body can be detected, then air passages must be cleared immediately. Remember Airways and Breathing.

Is victim bleeding?

Severe loss of blood will weaken the victim's condition and could cause death. The blood flow from a wound must be stopped, so that a blood clot can form. Learn the signs of internal bleeding and the correct treatment (*see page 41*). Remember Circulation.

Is victim unconscious?

Unconsciousness ranges from short fainting spells to deep coma. *It is not necessary to know all the degrees, but it is vital to note any changes in the state of alertness.* A deep coma can mean not breathing, and this must be treated first. Once the victim is breathing, put her into the recovery position (*see page 13*) to keep airway clear.

Remember ABC –
Airways, Breathing, Circulation.

CHECKING FOR BREATHING

The first priority
In the case of unconsciousness, you must establish that the casualty is breathing regularly before you can begin to treat injuries. This may involve artificial respiration (see page 13).

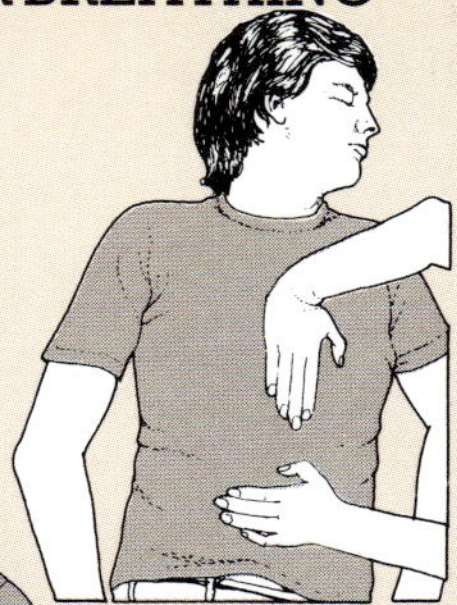

Feel chest & abdomen

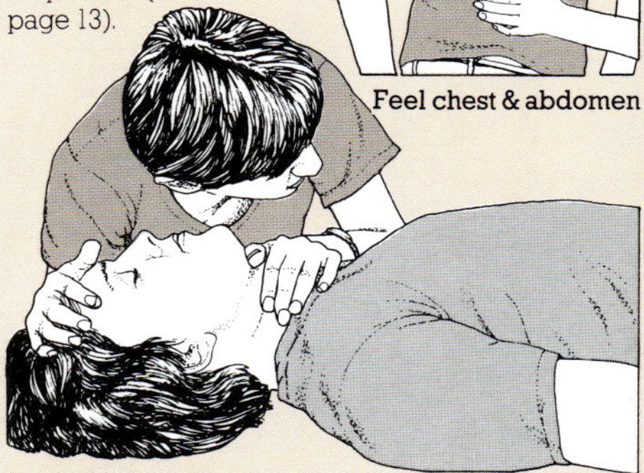

Listen for breathing

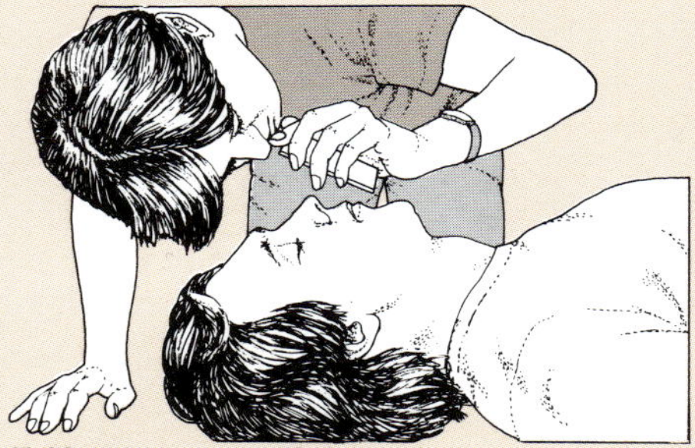

Hold a mirror to casualty's mouth

EMERGENCY ACTION IN CASE OF ACCIDENT

Procedure

- Go calmly to the scene, with a first aid kit, if available.
- Find out what has happened and the number of casualties.
- Decide who needs treatment first.
- Get a message to a doctor or ambulance, preferably by sending a helper.

Treatment priorities

- Remove the casualty from danger, or the danger from the casualty.
- Is the casualty breathing? If not, clear the airway and give artificial respiration. *(see page 13)*.
- Is the casualty bleeding? *(see page 39)*.
- Is the casualty unconscious?
- Examine for further injuries and treat. If the casualty is conscious, ask if he has pain and where.

Do's and don'ts

- *Do* continue to watch casualty's breathing.
- *Do* reassure casualty.
- *Do* record any change in casualty's condition.
- *Do* report any action taken, or treatment carried out, to ambulance crew or hospital.
- *Do* check for medic-alert cards or bracelets to indicate casualty's medical condition.
- *Do not* move badly-injured casualty.
- *Do not* take any unnecessary risks – you may become the next casualty.
- *Do not* delay vital medical treatment by dealing with minor injuries.
- *Do not* overheat the casualty – one blanket is sufficient cover.
- *Do not* give anything by mouth (except to burned casualties).

USING THE TELEPHONE IN AN EMERGENCY

1 Remain calm and patient.
2 Dial carefully to obtain the correct number quickly.
3 If you are dialling an operator controlled emergency services number, first tell the operator which service you require, e.g. fire, police, ambulance – or all three.
4 Give the operator the number of the telephone you are using in case you are disconnected.
5 When the emergency service answers, give the address or precise location of the place where help is required.
6 Tell them the nature of the emergency and be ready to give further information which may help.
7 Keep emergency telephone numbers close at hand – at home, they can be permanently displayed by the telephone *(see pages 92-3)*.

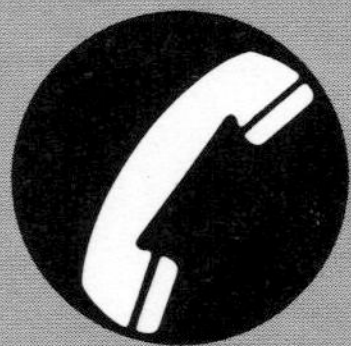

Speak clearly and precisely at all times.

Internal systems

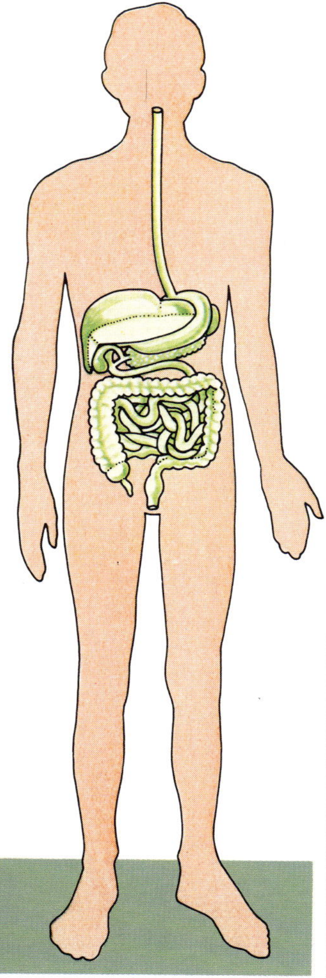

The digestive system
The digestive process is one in which the food we eat is broken down into energy giving and nutritious substances which can be absorbed by body tissue.

In order to run continuously as an efficient machine, the human body needs fuel to provide energy, and this comes from two sources: the food we eat and the air we breathe.

The food we eat is broken down by the *Digestive System* so that the nutritious content can be absorbed into the body tissues, and the waste products expelled by the excretory system.

The air we breathe through our *Respiratory System* contains life-giving oxygen. In the lungs, most of the oxygen is extracted and fed into the blood. Carbon dioxide is breathed out as waste.

In the *Circulatory System* the heart pumps the blood continuously through arteries to every part of the body. Nourishment and oxygen are absorbed by the body tissues and waste products are taken back into the blood which returns through veins to the heart, then to the lungs for a new supply of oxygen.

The *Nervous System* consists of the brain, which is the controlling centre, the spinal cord, which contains the nerve cells that carry messages to and from the brain, and a vast network of nerves throughout the body.

Circulatory system
The blood is the agent which carries the life-giving substances to all parts of the body.

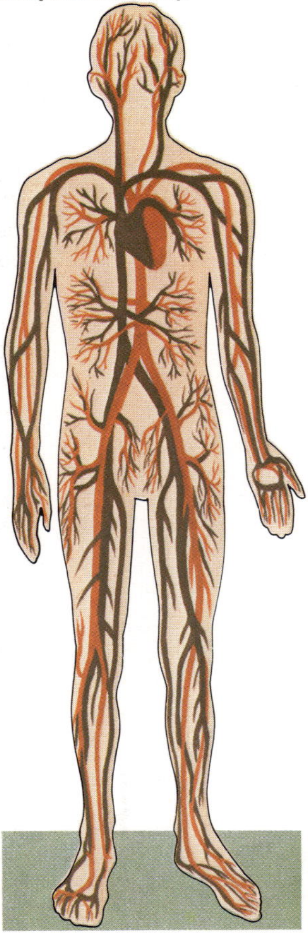

The respiratory system
The lungs feed the vital oxygen into the blood and eject unwanted carbondioxide.

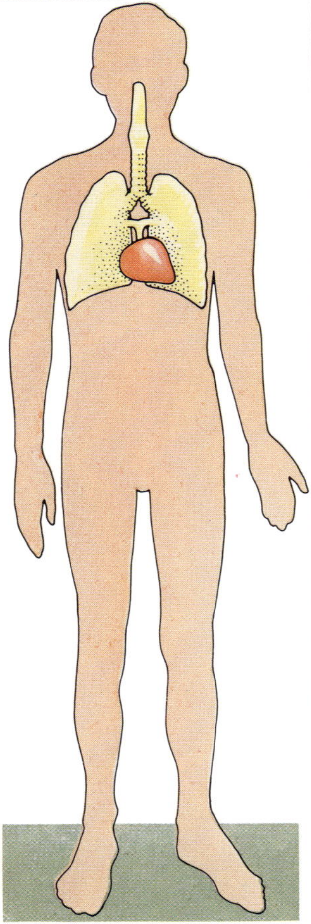

Nervous system
Information is carried to and from the brain by nerves, all of which are connected to the spinal cord.

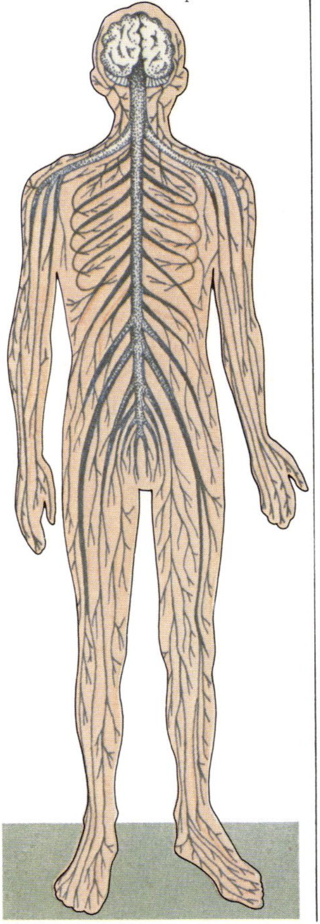

Casualty unconscious and not breathing

Remember, that in all emergencies where injury or illness occurs, the first priority for treatment is the casualty's breathing. The chart on this page sets out in precise order the steps that should be taken in dealing with a casualty whose breathing has stopped. Ideally, the procedure should be committed to memory, but carefully and accurately –

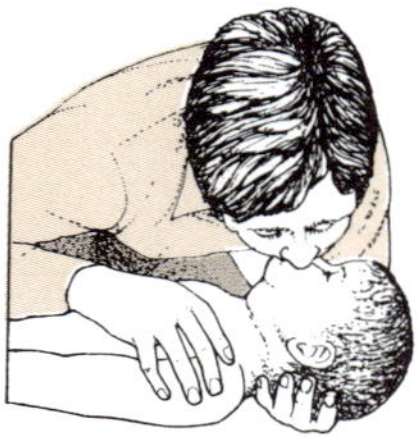

Babies/small children
For babies and young children it is best to blow into mouth and nose at the same time.

CLEARING THE AIRWAY

▶
Loosen clothing and clear the mouth
Lay the casualty on his back, if possible, and loosen clothing around throat, chest and waist. Using your finger, or a handkerchief, clear the mouth of loose debris: blood, dentures, etc.

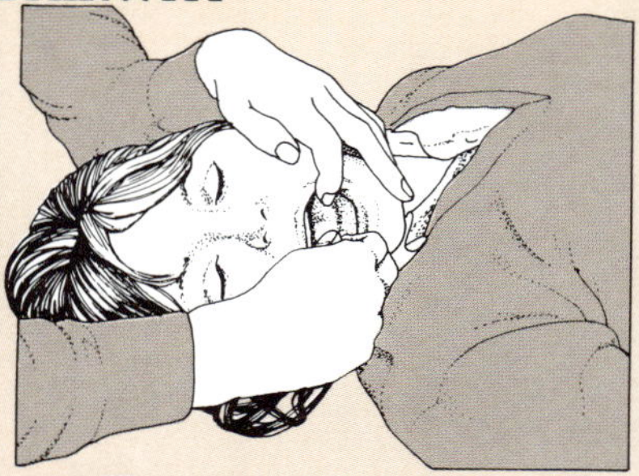

▶
Tilt head backwards and try to restart breathing
Tilt the head back as far as possible, while supporting the back of the neck with one hand. The nostrils should now be pointing upwards. Using your free hand, bring the lower jaw up to meet the upper jaw. If breathing does not restart, you must use artificial respiration.

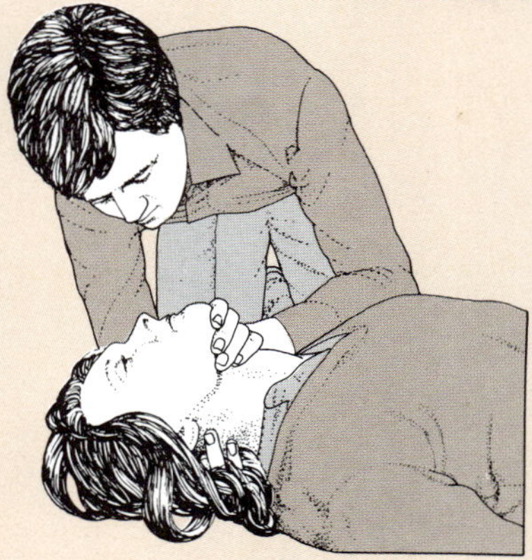

▶
Correct head position
When the nostrils point upwards, the tongue will not block the windpipe, and breathing may restart naturally.

Correct

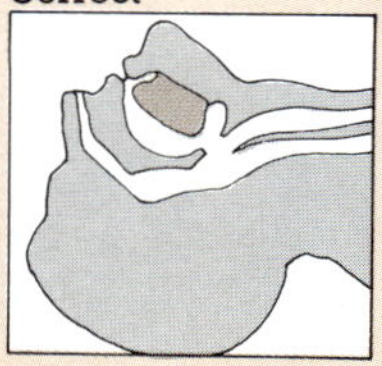

Incorrect

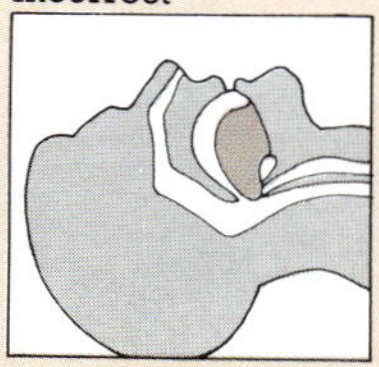

ARTIFICIAL RESPIRATION

Mouth-to-nose method
If the nose is not blocked, this method is preferable for adults. With the casualty's head tilted back and your free hand blocking his mouth, blow firmly into his nose. Watch his chest fall as the air leaves the lungs and blow again into his nose; do this rapidly 3 or 4 times, then repeat every 4/5 seconds until breathing restarts, or for about an hour.

Mouth-to-mouth
When using this method, pinch the casualty's nostrils and make sure that your lips form a seal around his mouth. Then proceed as above. When the casualty is breathing regularly, but still unconscious, he must be put into the recovery position.

NB When using either method of artificial respiration, remember to support the casualty's neck with one hand, and to watch for his chest rising as you blow into his lungs. If this does not happen, check again that the airway is clear.

Tilt head back to clear airway

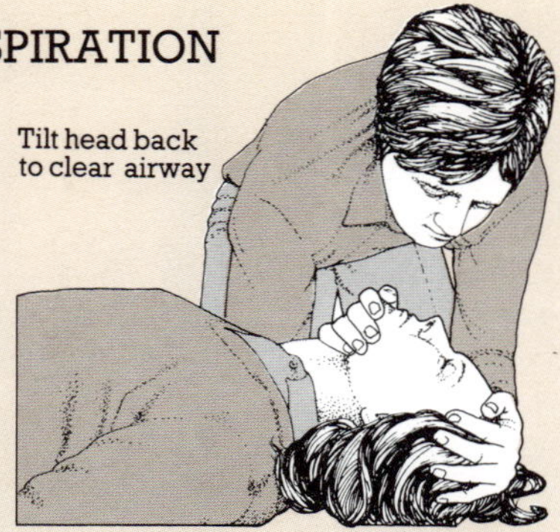

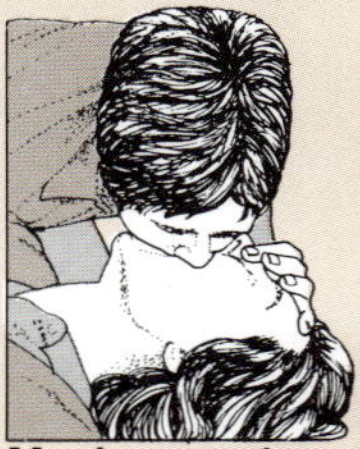

Mouth-to-mouth

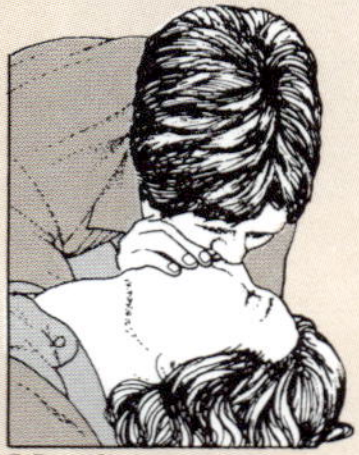

Mouth-to-nose

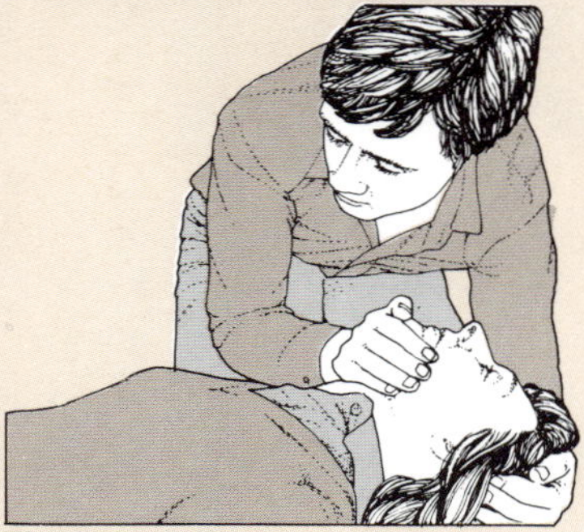

Watch chest fall

● *See opposite for babies and small children.*

Recovery positions

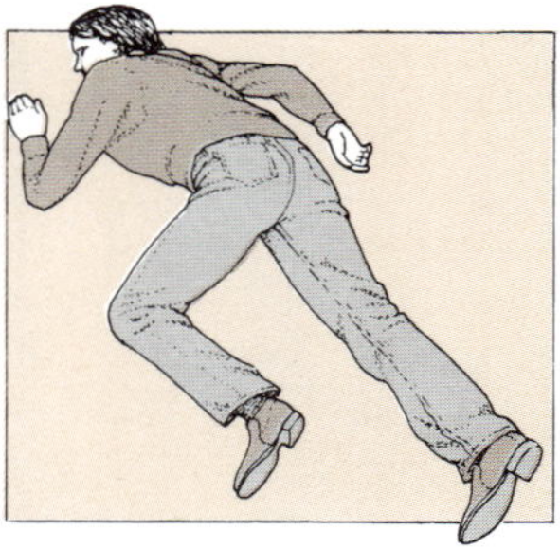

If the casualty is lying on the floor or ground

1. Place him, if possible, in face-down position.

2. Stand on one side of him, turn his head towards you, tilting it slightly backwards and move his jaw forwards so that his chin juts out and his tongue will not block the airway.

3. Pull up the arm and leg on the side that his head is facing, and bend them to form right angles. This will 'fix' his position.

●
See page 8 for 'Checking for breathing'.

First aid equipment

Basic equipment
A first aid kit need not be elaborate or expensive. Too much equipment can be a hindrance, but it is important that the contents are kept together in a portable, labelled container with a well-fitting lid. Items should be replaced when used, and the kit must be easily accessible but well out of the reach of young children. It is best kept separate from the household medicine chest.

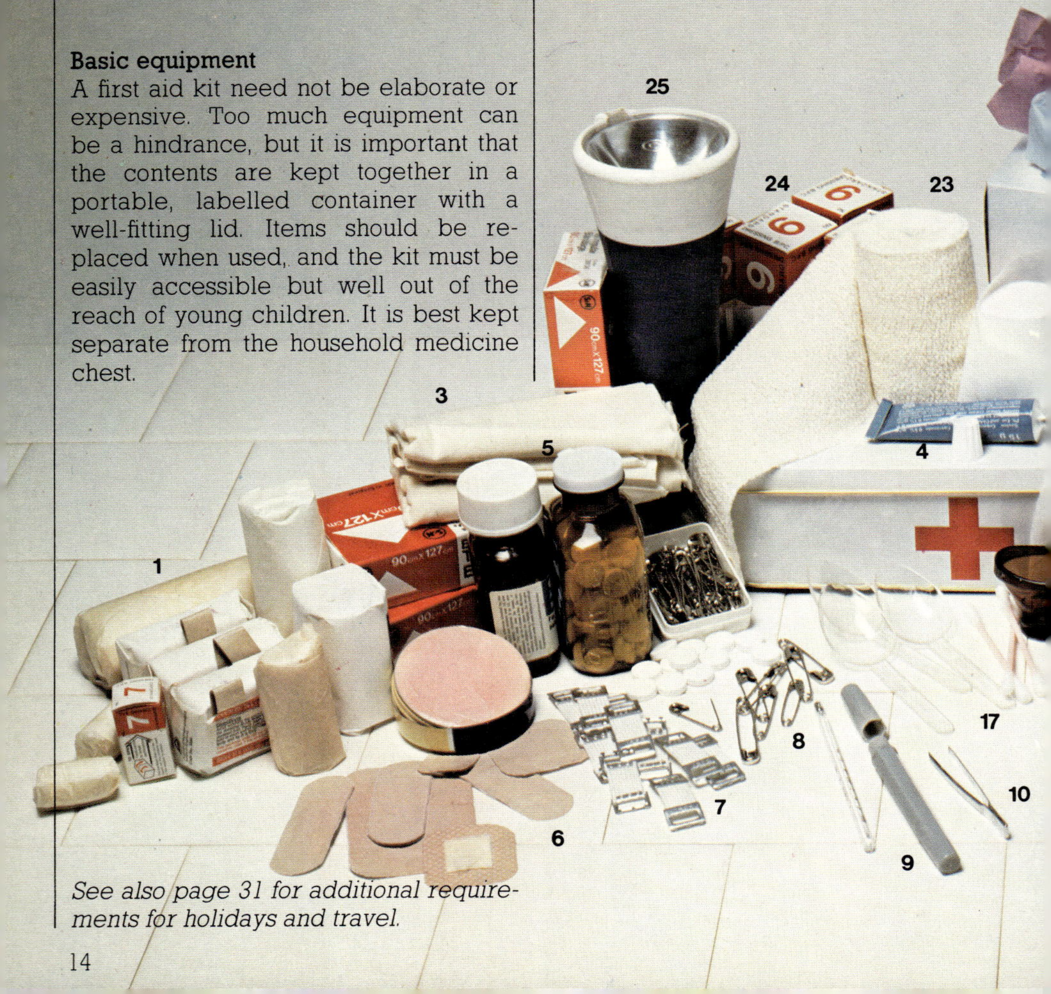

See also page 31 for additional requirements for holidays and travel.

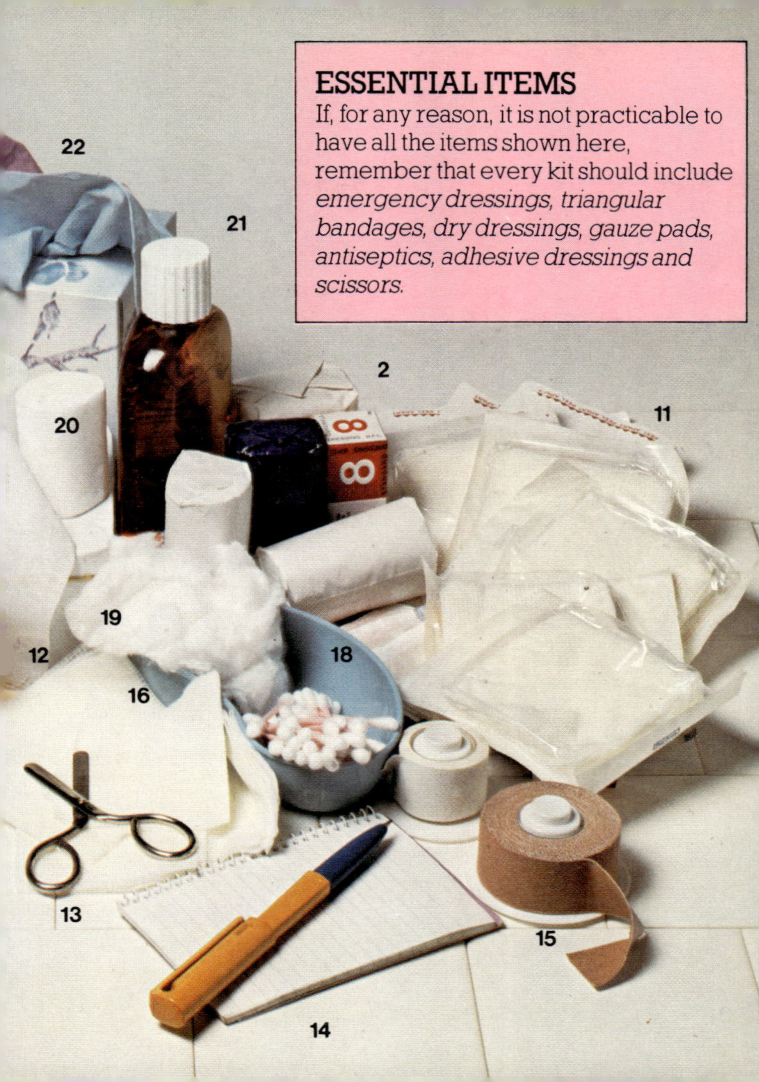

ESSENTIAL ITEMS

If, for any reason, it is not practicable to have all the items shown here, remember that every kit should include *emergency dressings, triangular bandages, dry dressings, gauze pads, antiseptics, adhesive dressings and scissors.*

First aid kit◀
Ideally, the domestic first aid kit should contain the following items:

1 Small emergency dressings (3 packs)
2 Medium emergency dressings (3 packs)
3 At least 4 triangular bandages
4 Antiseptic ointment
5 Mild pain killers
6 Assorted adhesive dressings
7 Bandage clips
8 Safety pins
9 Thermometer
10 Tweezers
11 Non adhesive dry dressings: 3 small, 3 large
12 Eyebath
13 Blunt ended scissors
14 Paper and pencil
15 Rolls of adhesive plaster
16 6 packs sterile gauze pads (7.5 cm square)
17 Cotton buds
18 Container for diluting antiseptic
19 Cotton wool
20 Cotton conforming bandages (3 x 5 cm, 3 x 7.5 cm)
21 Liquid antiseptic
22 Paper tissues
23 Crepe bandages (7.5 cm)
24 Large emergency dressings (3 packs)
25 Torch

Dressings

The First Aid kit should contain a selection of dressings. A dressing is put on a wound to prevent germs entering and causing infection, to help control bleeding, absorb any discharge and avoid further injury so that healing can take place.

Dressings should be sterile or packed under germ-free conditions because this will help healing. They must be porous, so that sweat will evaporate through them. (If the skin is moist, germ growth will be encouraged.)

Dressings should not be made of fluffy material, such as cotton wool, because this can leave stray fragments in the wound. If dressings have to be improvised in an emergency, use clean smooth material such as torn cotton sheets or handkerchiefs.

DRESSING A WOUND

When putting on a dressing keep everything as clean as possible, and always wash your hands before using any first aid equipment. Never cough or breathe over a wound, or touch the surface of the dressing to go on the wound.

TYPES OF DRESSING

EMERGENCY DRESSING

These are available in a range of sizes, usually with bandages attached. They are intended for use on large wounds. Extra padding can be placed over the dressing and bandaged into position.

DRY GAUZE DRESSINGS

These are primarily intended for use on small cuts and burns – provided that the area to be covered will not stick to the dressing and make removal painful.

NON-ADHESIVE DRESSINGS

These are recommended for covering areas which would stick to a dry gauze dressing – such as an extensive raw burn. They are available in most first aid kits.

ADHESIVE DRESSINGS

Useful only for very small cuts, they consist of absorbent pads with perforated adhesive backings.

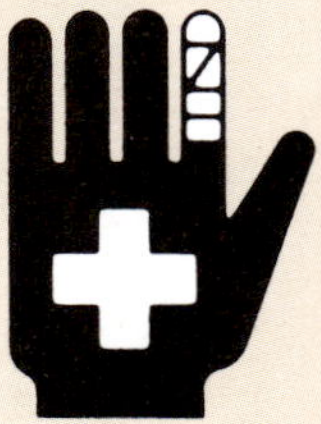

Bandages

A bandage is used to apply direct pressure over a dressing to control bleeding, keep dressings in place, restrict movement, and to provide support. Bandaging is not complicated. Modern conforming and crepe bandages stretch to the shape of the part being bandaged, and will hold dressings lightly but firmly in place, apply even pressure and will not loosen.

Triangular bandages can be bought, or made from linen or old cotton sheets by cutting a 90 cm (36 in.) square diagonally to form two bandages. They can be used as head or foot bandages, slings, and folded into narrow or broad bandages. Bandages can be improvised from scarves or towels.

An **Arm Sling** is used for injuries to ribs, upper arm and forearm, for a sitting or standing casualty. When applied, the arm should be comfortable, resting just above the belt line, with the wrist supported.

A **Triangular Sling** is used for injuries to the collar bone or the hand – when the forearm needs to be well-raised across the chest. An improvised sling can be made out of a headscarf, necktie or belt.

TRIANGULAR BANDAGES AND SLINGS

Folding a triangular bandage
Triangular bandages are extremely versatile, they can be used as slings, head bandages, narrow or broad bandages. Two folds, right, will form a broad bandage, three will make a narrow one.

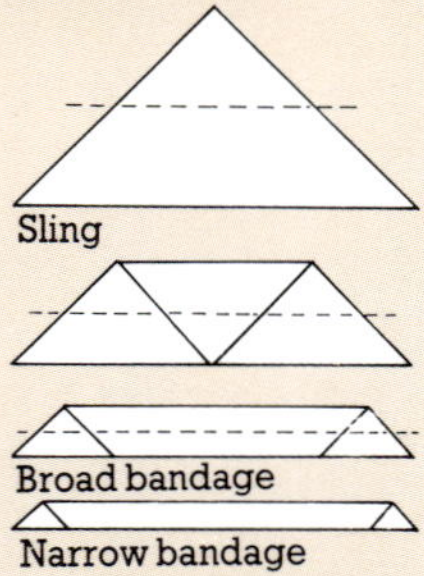

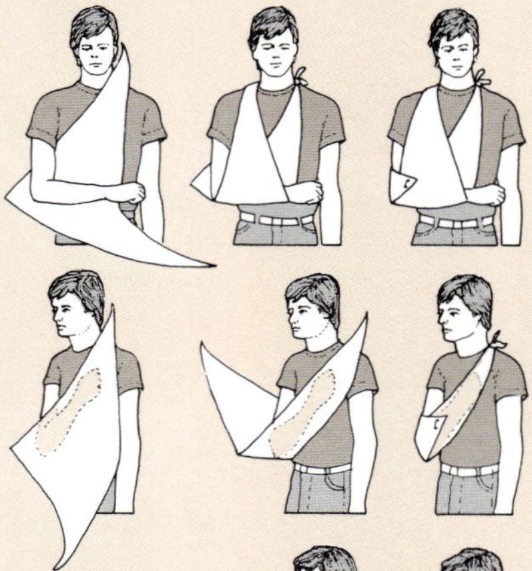

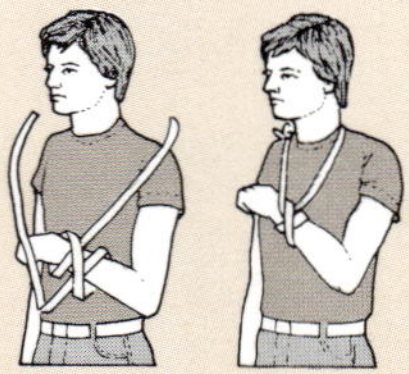

Making slings
The three stages of making slings: the arm sling, *top*, and the triangular sling, *below*. A collar and cuff sling is shown, *right*.

MOTORCYCLE SAFETY

Motorcyclists run a very high risk of involvement in an accident. To reduce the risk, always ride with your lights on – in daylight as well – and wear a good quality helmet.

Full-face helmets▸
Make sure that the visor is well-made and will not mist or scratch easily.

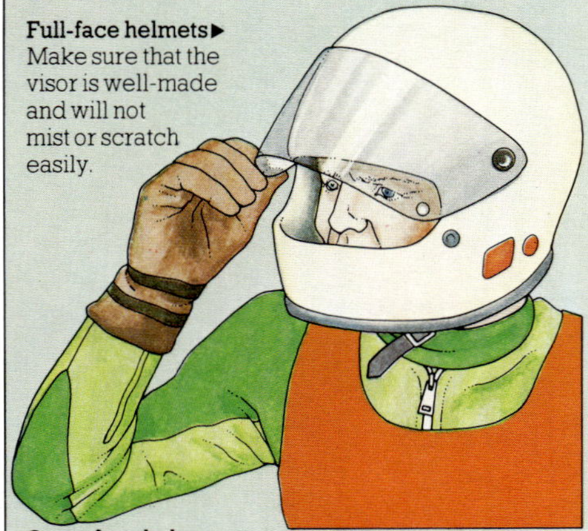

Open-face helmets▾
These can be used with goggles or visors. Make sure the chinstrap is soundly made.

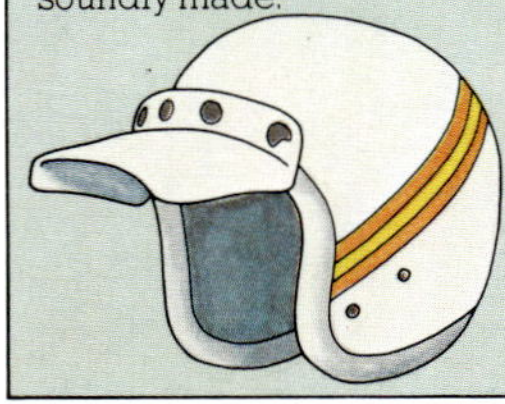

● **Choosing a helmet**
Make sure that your helmet fits snugly and securely; that the chinstrap is firm and comfortable and that the general construction of the helmet is strong. Always look for an official seal of approval for safety.

Accident prevention

Even though the cause of an accident may appear to be faulty apparatus, or poor weather conditions, underlying this may be someone's thoughtlessness or carelessness in not observing the simple rules of commonsense. And often it is the innocent – the very young or the very old – who are the victims, not the culprit.

Well-maintained homes will prevent many accidents. So will teaching the whole family to swim, and to know the dangers of different waterways. If youngsters keep to their road drill and are educated in road safety, they will respond to the dangers of traffic. Motorists always wearing seat-belts (even on the shortest journey), young children strapped into special seats on the back seat of a car, motor-cyclists wearing crash-helmets – all will certainly *help* to avoid serious, even fatal, injuries.

Outdoor and holiday activities are bound to have their risks. To avoid the unnecessary ones, don't over-do things – whether it's overstraining the body by playing a game when you are tired or 'out of condition', or lying too long in the unaccustomed hot sunshine on a foreign beach.

Safety for road users
Cyclists can improve their safety rating by attending proficiency courses and by wearing special fluorescent jackets.

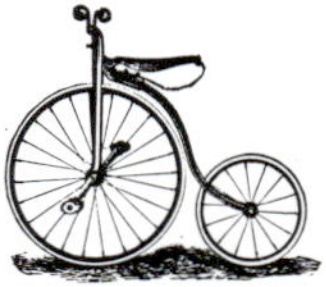

Pedestrians, *right*, should always be conscious of safety drill and children should be properly instructed. Seat belts and head restraints, *below*, greatly reduce the risk of injury in motor accidents.

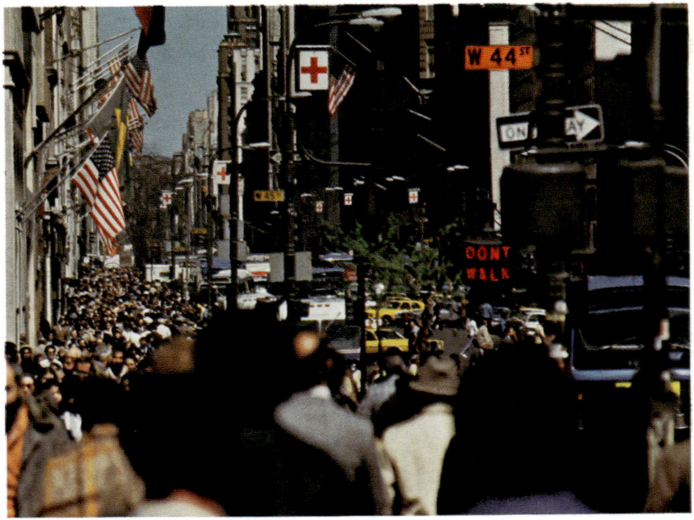

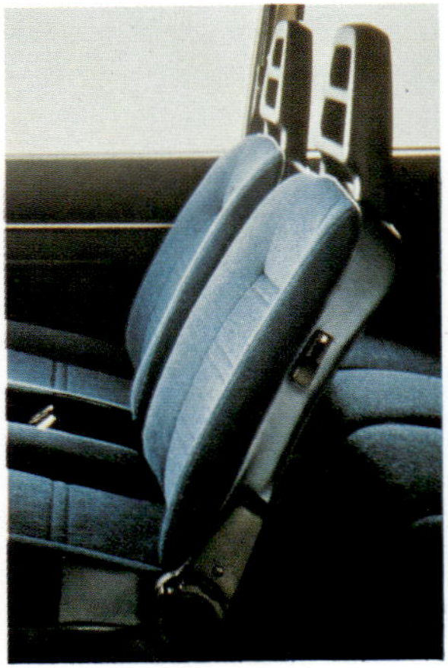

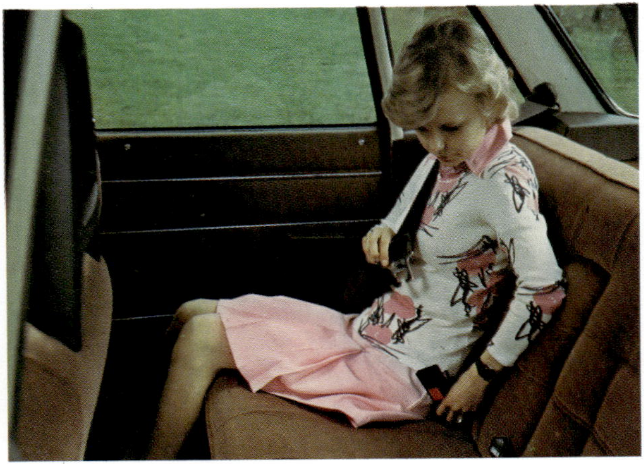

Think safety

'Thinking Safety' is essential, not just to avoid accidents to ourselves, but also to safeguard those unable to see possible dangers. Acting safely can be just as much a habit as taking risks, but it does, initially, involve conscious effort.

Road Accidents

A very high proportion of all accidental deaths occur on the roads. Care is needed if you are walking along a road because almost as many pedestrians as car users are killed. Road junctions in towns and country roads are the worst accident sites.

Prevention of many such accidents is possible by reducing speeds, improving roads, not drinking and driving, keeping the vehicle well serviced and driving according to the weather conditions. But, most of the pedestrians killed are aged betweeen 5 and 9 years; most cyclists killed or injured are between 10 and 14. The greatest number of casualties among car drivers occur at ages 18 and 19, for motor-cyclists at 17 and for moped users at 16. Every year, more people are on the roads – so 'thinking safety' must include early education on the rules of using the road.

Sporting Activities

All sports have dangers. Those that are an intrinsic part of the game can result in knee injuries (common to many sports), broken bones or pulled muscles. The professional knows these dangers and is ready to meet them by keeping in good physical condition, wearing correct clothing and equipment – and by using common-sense.

The enthusiastic amateur, however, does not always follow this example by knowing and observing these basic rules. So, by not 'thinking safety' he adds unnecessary risks to the game. One instance shown by this lack of forethought is that British surgeons report hundreds of eye injuries among squash players who do not wear the recommended eye protectors. The effect of the impact of a squash ball is like a rubber bullet – it can burst the eyeball.

Swimming causes seven times more deaths than any other recreation. More than 600 deaths from drowning are reported every year. Most victims are children, and drowning occurs through thoughtlessness, – not just in the sea and swimming pools, but also in canals, rivers, quarries and garden pools.

OUTDOOR SAFETY	Do's	Don'ts
ON THE ROAD 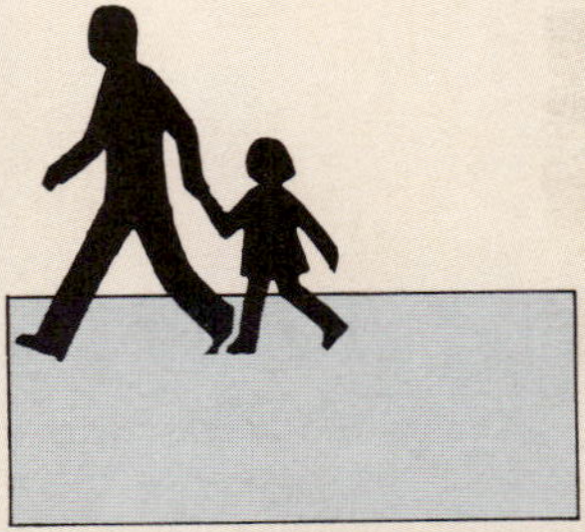	**Pedestrians** – wear reflective clothing at night. **Cyclists** – wear reflective clothing at night and make sure the cycle has good front and rear lighting. **Pedestrians** – face the oncoming traffic where there is no sidewalk.	Forget to wear your safety belt or crash helmet. Let small children sit in the front seat – even on an adult passenger's lap. Let children ride bicycles without proper road safety instruction. Neglect the condition of vehicles.
ON THE SPORTS FIELD 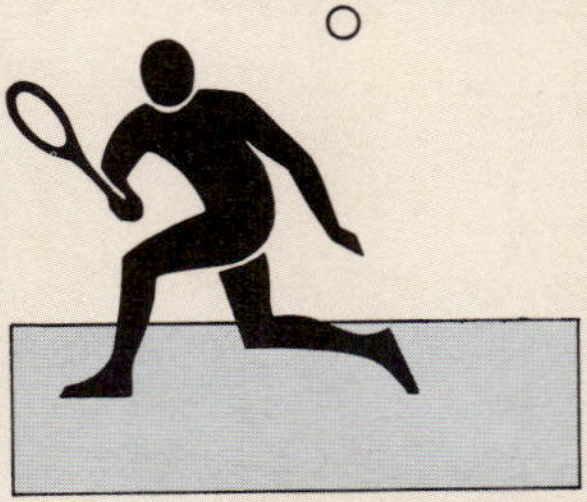	Always wear the correct protective clothing. Make sure that your equipment is in good condition and working properly. Warm up before a game – cold muscles are liable to injury.	Take part in games if you are not fit – or if you are suffering from an injury. Continue to play when fatigued. Attempt the impossible – or something you have not prepared for.
ON AND IN WATER 	See that all the family learn to swim and basic rescue methods. Obey all warning notices about bathing, currents, etc.	Let children play in boats without adults present. Let young children bathe without supervision.

The safe house

We may think that home is a safe place, but in most industrialised countries almost as many people die from accidents in the home as on the roads. Most at risk are the very young and the very old.
Falls and fires cause most accidental deaths in the home. Other frequent causes include poisoning and suffocation. But very many home accidents, especially in the kitchen and bathroom, can be prevented by continuous care and thought. Always have permanent gas and electrical appliances installed by qualified fitters, and buy only those appliances that carry official safety symbols. Remember that water conducts electricity, and never touch a switch or appliance if your hands are wet.

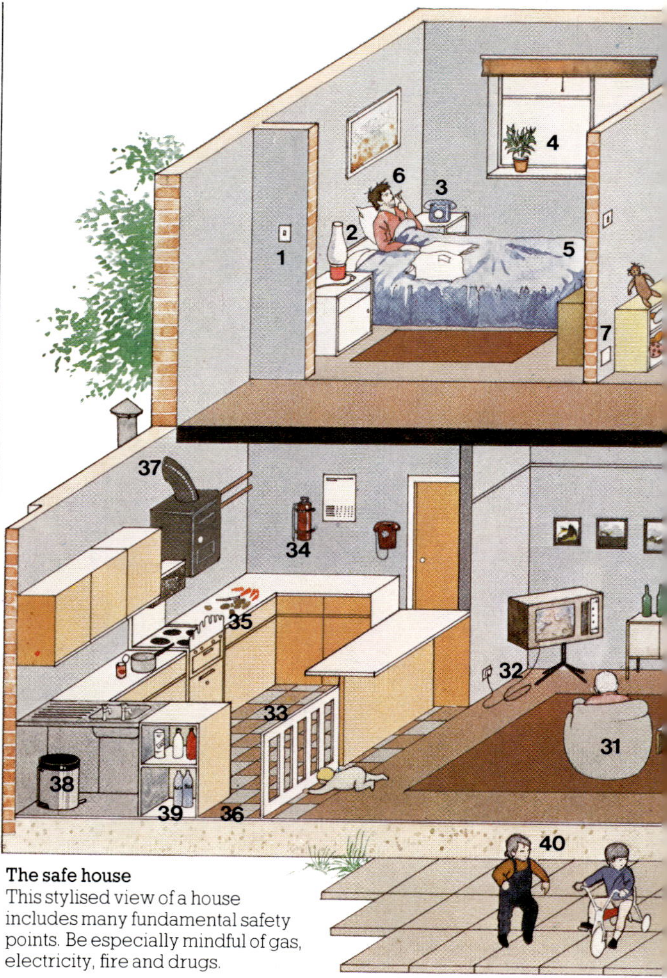

The safe house
This stylised view of a house includes many fundamental safety points. Be especially mindful of gas, electricity, fire and drugs.

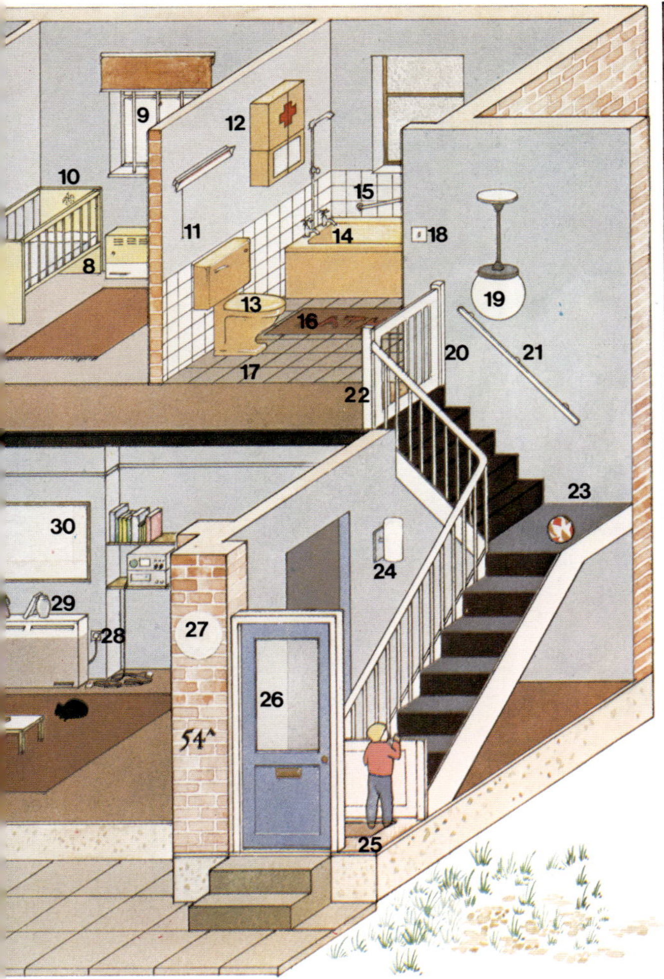

SAFETY INDOORS

1 Adequate lighting for passageways
2 Access to main light from bed
3 Telephone in upstairs room
4 Escape facility from upstairs
5 Keep electric blankets/heaters in good order
6 Never smoke in bed
7 Safety covers on electric outlets
8 High sided cots No pillows
9 Safety bars on windows
10 No lead paint on furniture
11 Cord switches on heaters
12 High level storage of drugs
13 Scrupulous hygiene in w.c.
14 Non-slip mats in bath
15 Hand rails for elderly
16 Non-slip mats on floors
17 Hygienic floor coverings
18 Access to stairs light switch
19 Adequate lighting for stairs
20 Safety gates on stairs
21/22 Secure handrails
23 Secure carpets/ No obstruction
24 Adequate lighting in hall
25 No rugs on polished floors
26 Laminated glass in doors
27 Adequate light for entrance
28 Safe wiring and connections
29 No objects on heaters
30 No mirrors above 'live' heaters
31 Safe materials for furnishings
32 No trailing electrical flex
33 Safety gate to kitchen
34 Fire extinguisher in kitchen
35 Guards around stove/cooker
36 Non-slip floor coverings
37 Ventilation for gas units
38 Hygienic waste can/fitted lid
39 Cleaning materials locked, or kept out of children's reach
40 Play area visible from house

Safety in the home

The most expensive purchase in a lifetime for the majority of people is their home. Much time and money is spent in choosing the right furnishings, carpets and appliances.

A careful motorist ensures his car's good running by regular servicing. We depend on similar care being taken when we use public transport. So it is just as important to check regularly the continuing safety of our home.

Modern homes contain a lot of electrical and gas appliances, perhaps open fires, furniture with inflammable stuffing, poisons in the form of drugs and medicines, as well as insecticides, weed-killers, household bleaches, liquid fuels – the list of lethal possibilities is endless. All must be treated with care.

Do not think that a flame is needed to start a fire. Burnable material will burst into flames spontaneously if it gets hot enough. If you want free expert advice about fire hazards in your home, you can obtain it from the Fire Prevention Officer at your local Fire Brigade Headquarters. Have the house-wiring circuit checked every five years. If your wiring is more than 25 years old, it may well need renewing.

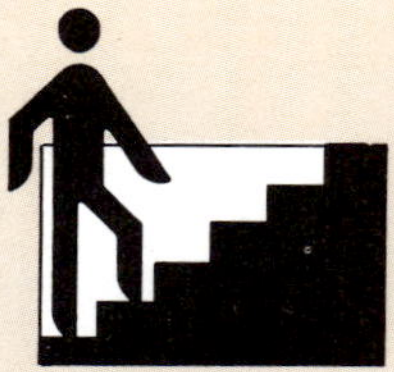

TO PREVENT FALLS

- Have adequate lighting at house entrance.
- Have two-way light switches on stairs and landings.
- Have safety gates at top and foot of stairs for children.
- Make sure that hand rails and bannisters are secure.
- Make sure that stair rods are firmly fixed.
- Have non-slip backing on rugs.
- Do not leave toys and other objects lying on floors and stairs.
- Do not have door handles that can get caught in clothing.
- When a child is in a cot, make sure that the side is up and firmly fixed.
- Make sure that children cannot climb through open windows.

TO PREVENT FIRES

- Have guards around all fires and heaters.
- Fill oil heaters out of doors.
- Unplug electrical appliances after use.
- Keep all appliances in good repair and use according to the instructions.
- Have a fire extinguisher installed in the kitchen.
- Do not leave matches or lighters where children can reach them.
- Do not smoke in bed.
- Do not stand oil heaters in draughts or where they could be knocked over.
- Do not carry lighted oil heaters. Do not use aerosol sprays near fires or naked flames.
- Do not overload the electrical circuit.
- Do not leave petrol cans where there may be sparks or naked flames.

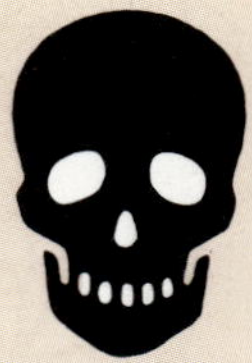

TO PREVENT POISONING

- Keep all medicines and drugs in labelled containers out of reach of children.
- When taking medicines, check the correct dosage first.
- All surplus and used medicines should be thrown away. You can flush them down the toilet or return them to the pharmacist.
- Do not take drugs or medicines in front of your children.
- Do not leave tablets in handbags or attaché cases.
- Do not leave sleeping tablets beside the bed or take tablets when drowsy or in the dark.
- Do not take sleeping tablets or drugs before a hot bath.
- Do not keep domestic chemicals where children can reach them, including dishwater detergents.

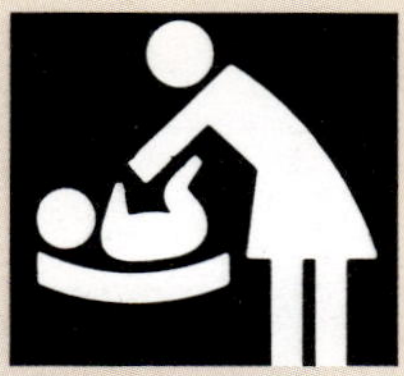

TO PREVENT ASPHYXIATION

- Always stay with a baby while feeding from bottle – in case of choking.
- Always pat the baby's back after feeding, to bring up wind and avoid inhalation of food.
- Keep all plastic bags out of children's reach.
- Have adequate ventilation for all gas fires and stoves.
- Keep all air vents and grills clear.
- Do not give a small baby a pillow in a cot or carriage.
- Do not use plastic bags or sheeting as a waterproof covering for mattresses.
- Do not use spray guns or chemicals where there is not adequate ventilation.
- Do not run a vehicle engines with garage door shut.
- Never put a baby to sleep on her front.

FIRST AID IF CLOTHING IS ON FIRE

Pull victim to ground
A person whose clothing is on fire must be prevented from standing or moving about – or the flames will rapidly spread. Use force if necessary, to get the victim to the ground.

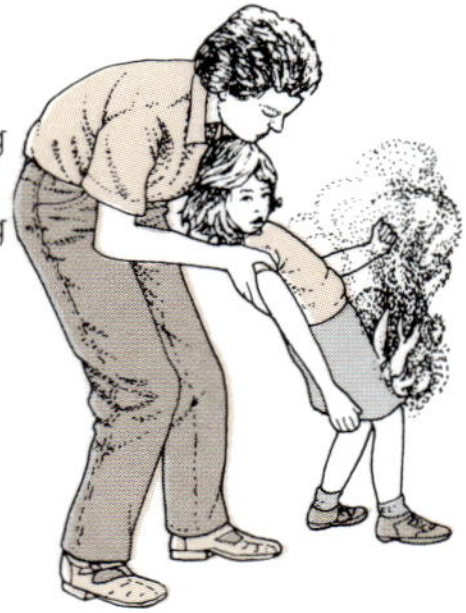

Extinguish flames
Use a blanket, rug or any heavy cloth (but no nylon or other synthetic materials) to smother the flames. Hold the material in front of you as you approach the victim.

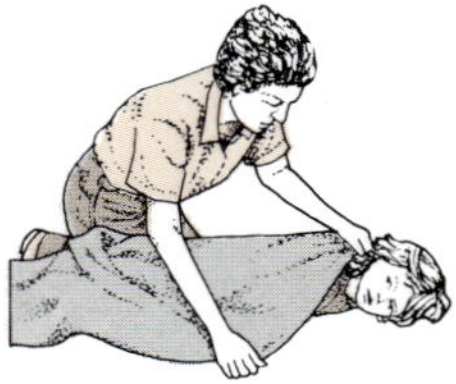

Cool burned areas
Cool the victim's burns with gently running cool water for at least ten minutes. Do not apply any pressure to burnt skin. Give a small amount to drink to **conscious** victims.

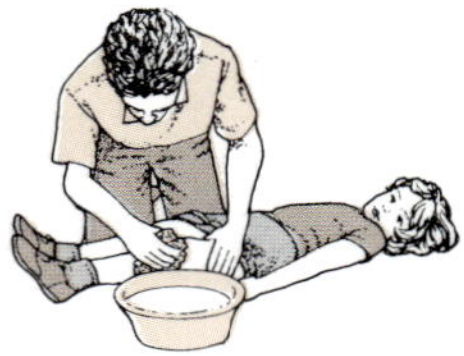

Give reassurance
Make the victim as comfortable as possible and offer plenty of reassurance. If the burns are serious, call an ambulance. Minor burns can be treated at home (*see page 76*).

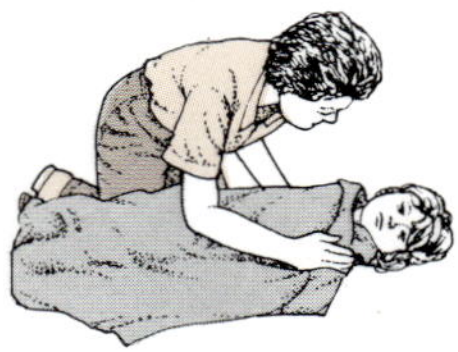

The safe garden

Just as your home should be made safe to avoid accidents, care is also needed outside. Garages and garden sheds are often the storeplaces of dangerous materials. It is very easy to leave the odd tool lying around, or to put off repairing the broken path, but an accident can happen before you realize what caused it.

1 Rubbish/refuse
Put it in bags and take it away – before children start getting rusty nails in their feet.

2 Bonfires
Keep bonfires away from buildings, trees and fences and safely contained in an incinerator. Supervise children near bonfires.

3 Lawnmowers
If you value your fingers – don't tamper with them. Switch off power or engine before attempting repair work.

4 Frames and cloches
Make sure that they are clearly visible and not hidden by shrubs or weeds. Plastic frames are safest.

5 Discarded tools
Don't leave tools lying around – they cause a surprisingly high number of accidents.

6 Chemicals/poisons
Store out of the reach of children. Label containers clearly and do not use old drink bottles.

7 Ponds/pools
Keep them shallow and do not let children play unattended near them.

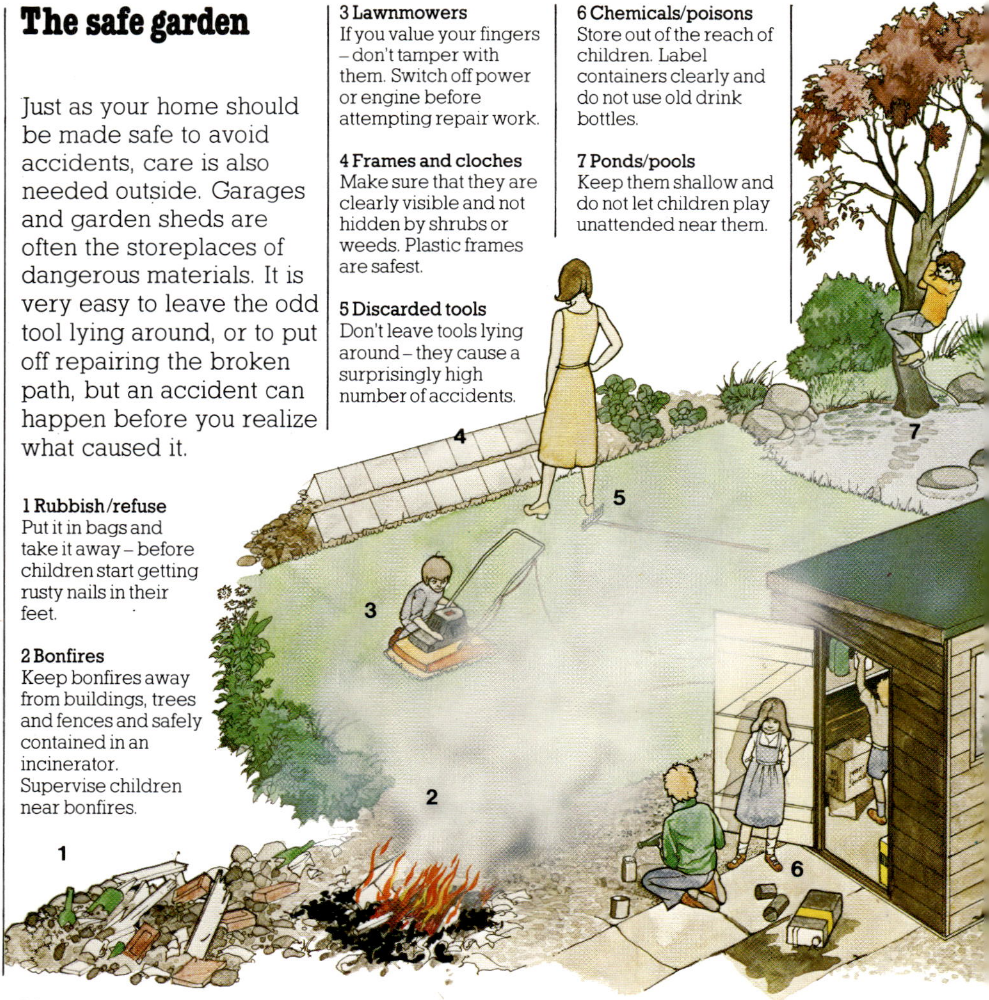

8 Glass/glazing
Remove and replace broken glass immediately – this applies to garden frames and cloches too.

9 Tool storage
A proper storing place for tools will discourage carelessness – and the tools are less likely to be put to the wrong use.

10 Vehicles
Take care when reversing – you may not see young children or animals.

11 Paths and steps
Keep them in good repair. Loose paving and broken steps cause many falls.

12 Overhead safety
Attend to loose tiles immediately. Make sure that your ladder is secure and in good repair. Do not attempt to reach too far.

13 Hygiene
Keep drains and refuse containers clean and sealed.

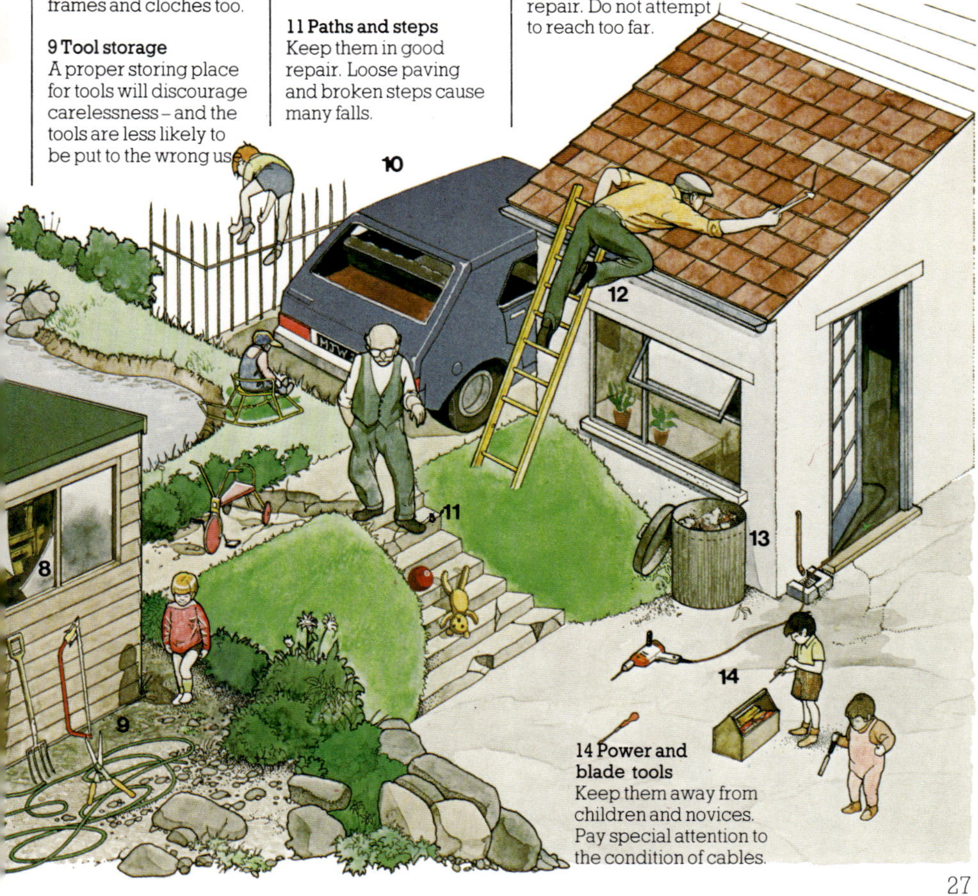

14 Power and blade tools
Keep them away from children and novices. Pay special attention to the condition of cables.

WHEN TO SEEK MEDICAL ADVICE

- Always, if the casualty has been unconscious – even if only for a short period.
- If bleeding is persistent, or if a wound needs stitching.
- If there is a possibility of infection. Perhaps from a deep knife wound, penetration by a nail, or where there is dirt or a foreign body in the wound.
- After bites or deep scratches from animals.
- If a child has swallowed a sharp object, e.g. an open safety pin.
- Following muscular strain, bruises, sprains, or black eyes – there may be further injury.
- Where the face or eyelids are burned, or where any burned surface area exceeds more than about 2.5cm (1in) square (after cooling treatment has been given at home).
- Where the casualty's condition following a minor injury does not improve after a few days.
- When young children have stomach upsets and lose body fluid through diarrhoea and vomiting. This is particularly important in hot weather or unfamiliar climates.

Home treatment/self help

Home treatment

'Home treatment' means treatment which is adequate to deal with minor injuries and ailments, without medical aid.

But it is important to recognize what is considered 'minor', when home treatment *is* sufficient, and when a doctor should be consulted.

As mothers of young children know, small cuts and scratches can occur daily – so can accidental burns in the kitchen. Most mishaps will be minor, and curing or healing take place without complications – provided attention is given at once.

At home, it is worthwhile to keep a list of emergency numbers by your telephone: your doctor and dentist, electricity and gas companies, the fire brigade, nearby friends and relatives.

Self help

Self-help is the first aid you can give yourself after being taken ill, or after an accident has occurred while alone, either at home or outside.

More and more people, especially the elderly, live alone. Following a fall, it may be some time before anyone comes by. But in such circumstances, provided you remain calm, you can help your condition considerably. In fact, any self-help given at this time may well assist the treatment given later by a doctor or hospital.

After a fall, or after being taken ill, try not to panic. Work out what might have happened, and what injury you have. Are you bleeding? Do you think any bones are broken? Now what can you do?

If you are elderly, and you fall suddenly, lie still for a few moments to get your breath back before trying to rise.

If you are bleeding, apply pressure with your fingers to stop the flow of blood. Raise the affected part, if possible, and tie a handkerchief or scarf over the wound.

If you think a leg might be broken, try to prop it up on a cushion or folded garment, so that the limb is supported. If an arm is injured, hold it with the other arm.

If you feel faint, loosen clothing around your neck and waist, breathe deeply. Take out any dentures and, if you can, get into the recovery position (*p. 13*). Or, sit with your head between your knees. After a few moments, you may feel much better.

If you are at home, and can reach the telephone, dial for help. Or knock on a wall so that someone can help you. Get into the most comfortable position to lessen pain until help arrives. Pull a garment around you so that you will not get cold.

All this may seem optimistic. If you fall suddenly, the tendency is to panic. But if you can keep calm, and remember the priorities of first aid as you would when treating someone else, it will help your condition.

Der Doctor.

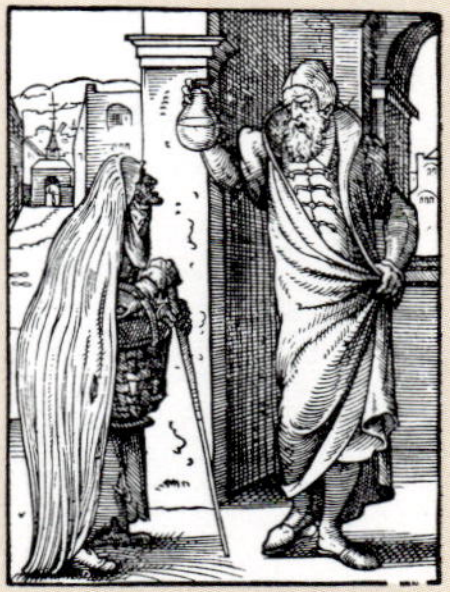

Ich bin ein Doctor der Artzney/
An dem Harn kan ich ſehen frey
Was kranckheit ein Menſchn thut beladn
Dem kan ich helffen mit Gotts gnadn
Durch ein Syrup oder Recept
Das ſeiner kranckheit widerſtrebt/
Daß der Menſch wider werd geſund/
Arabo die Artzney erfund.

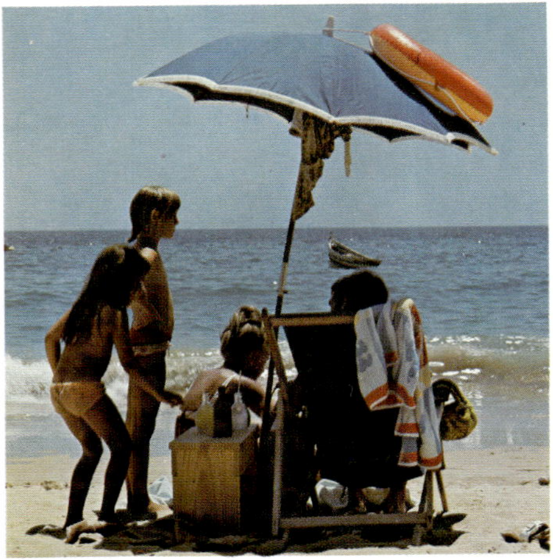

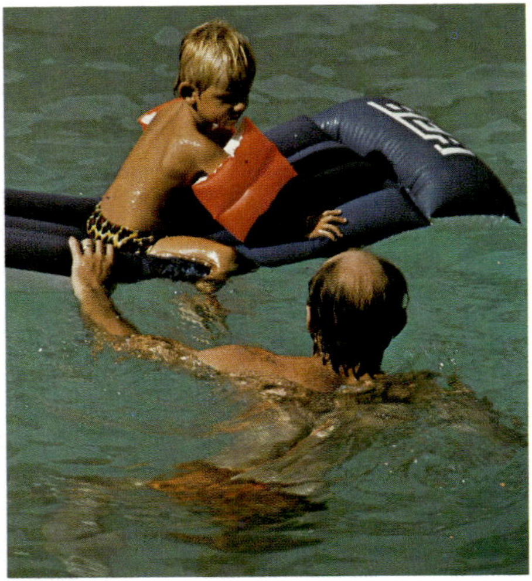

Holidays and travel

Organised activities, such as school sports, usually make arrangements for First Aid. But for family outings and vacations (when you may be out of reach of medical aid), it is worth being prepared for emergencies.

Travel sickness can spoil journeys: there are many safe ways of avoiding this, including sea-bands, which press on acupressure points on your wrist to prevent nausea. See your pharmacist.

Soothing creams can help irritation from heat spot, rashes, insect stings and mosquito bites – Calendula and Calamine are good choices. Sunscreens are essential – the higher the factor number, the better. Look out for those which block UVA and UVB rays. Bring along some insect repellent.

Be ready to treat bleeding from cuts or minor wounds from seaside rocks, or sea urchins (wear gloves to remove spikes). If you are staying in a hot climate, get used to the unaccustomed heat gradually. Take sensible precautions and learn to recognise signs of heat exhaustion. Stomach upsets caused by allergies or mild food poisoning usually respond to rest and 24 hours of fluids only.

Sun and sea

Sunshine and water are essential ingredients of most vacations. Both, however, are capable of spoiling them, unless sensible precautions are taken. Many holidays are ruined by sunburn achieved on the first day. Get used to the sun gradually, and always wear a protective sunscreen with a high factor number. Bathing in the sea can be dangerous, especially for children – even if they are good swimmers. Parents should supervise them and make sure that younger children wear life-preservers.

Holiday extras

In addition to the items shown on page 14/15, those shown here will be valuable on vacation – or while travelling.

1 water sterilisation tablets
2 insect repellent cream
3 antiseptic wipes
4 soothing lotion for sunburn
5 high factor sunscreen
6 insect spray
7 antiseptic cream
8 mild painkillers
9 antiseptic ointment
10 assorted adhesive plasters

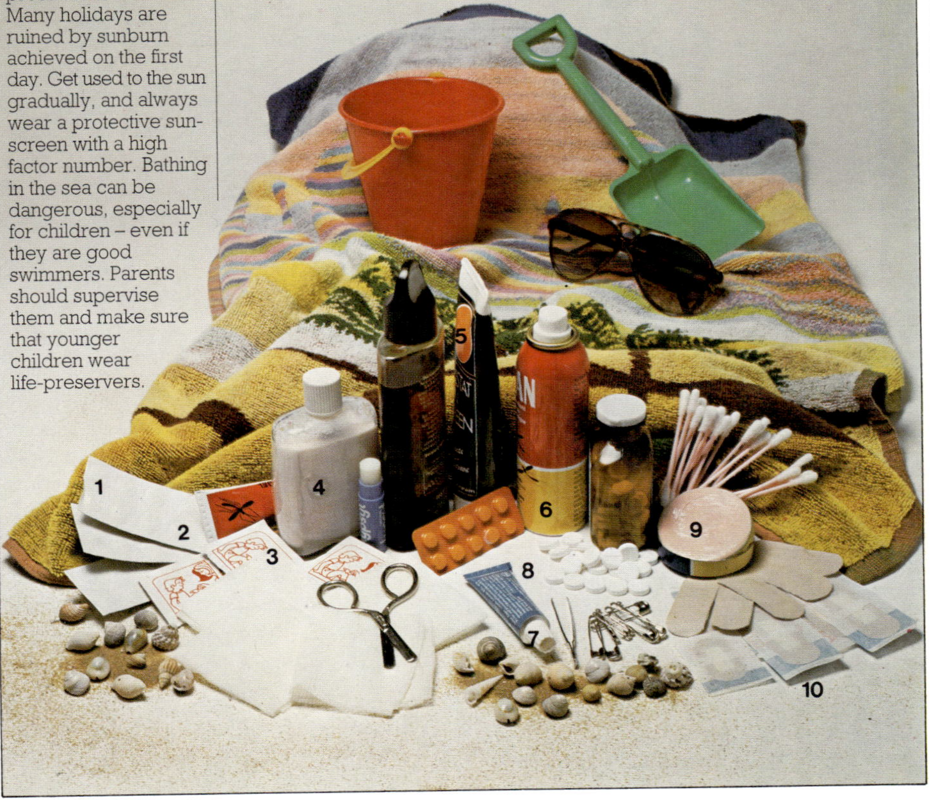

Remember ABC – Airways, Breathing, Circulation.

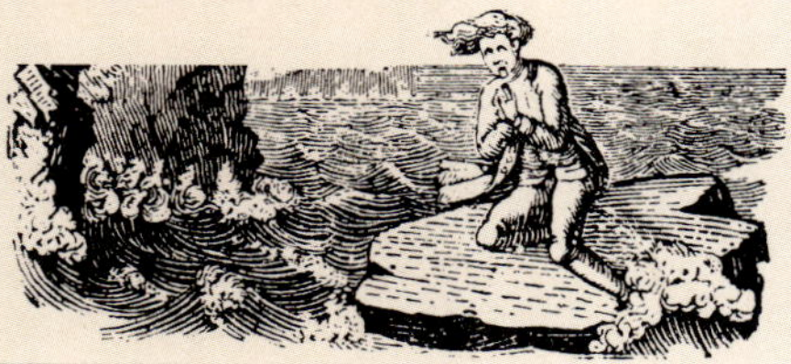

Basic rules & priorities

Everyone should be capable of helping to save a life in an emergency. Most of us have a smattering of knowledge, but lack the confidence to apply it, fearing that we may not do the right thing.

If you can memorise the few basic rules and priorities and practise the routines, you will gain confidence – and be able to do everything in your power to help a victim.

First: remove the victim from further danger, or danger from the victim. *Now*: check his airways. Is he breathing? Is he bleeding? Is he unconscious? Treat these conditions first.

Don't overheat a victim: one blanket is always enough covering. Do not give anything at all by mouth (unless she is a conscious burn victim, and then a small quantity of fluid is appropriate). Never leave an unconscious person unattended. Ensure the victim sees a doctor or goes to hospital after First Aid treatment.

The method given here for artificial respiration is by breathing directly into a person's lungs. The chest compression/expansion methods by external pressure require training and should only be given by expert personnel.

Breathing

Normal breathing is regular and quiet, but when breathing is difficult, it can be noisy, cause frothing at the mouth and nose and, possibly, blueness of the lips and ears (indicating that not enough oxygen is being supplied).
If a person stops breathing, he becomes unconscious because of inadequate oxygenation of tissue, in particular of brain cells. The failure to breathe may be due to a blocked airway, in which case the blockage must be removed (*p. 12/13*).
But there are many other possible causes of failure to breathe, and if a blocked airway is not the cause, then artificial respiration must be given at once. In all cases the treatment is the same and must be given immediately until the casualty can receive medical aid. **If breathing stops, death can occur within a few minutes.**
When we breathe in, air containing oxygen is drawn into the lungs as the chest expands. The lungs consist of many small tubes and tiny air sacs. Oxygen passes from these air sacs into blood vessels.
When we breathe out, the chest contracts, compresses the lungs and sends up gas contents (waste products from the blood) back into the air. In this way, carbon dioxide is expelled from the body, but there is still oxygen (16 per cent) in the air breathed out. When giving artificial respiration by breathing into a person's lungs, your breath holds enough oxygen to help re-start his breathing.

N.B.

If breathing has stopped, give treatment immediately:

- **Check for breathing** *see page eight*
- **Clear blocked airway** *see page twelve*
- **Apply artificial respiration** *see page thirteen*
- **Place casualty in recovery position** *see page thirteen*
- **Seek qualified medical help** *send someone for help immediately*

Choking/Drowning

Choking	Choking can occur when food "goes down the wrong way" or if a child puts a large object in his mouth. He may cough, which can help to clear the obstruction, but if not, treatment is essential.
Treatment for choking	Try to hook the obstruction in the throat with a finger. Help to remove the object by giving three or four sharp blows on the back between the shoulder blades. A small child can be held upside down. If breathing stops, clear airway and give artificial respiration (p. 13).
Drowning	Drowning occurs when water prevents air from entering the lungs, and breathing stops. Start treatment as soon as the victim's head is clear of the water.
Treatment for drowning	See that the airway is clear. Give artificial respiration (p. 13) for up to an hour if necessary. If breathing starts regularly, put the victim in the recovery position (p. 13). Watch in case further artificial respiration is needed.

HEIMLICH MANOEUVRE

(Abdominal Thrust method) is a highly effective treatment for choking

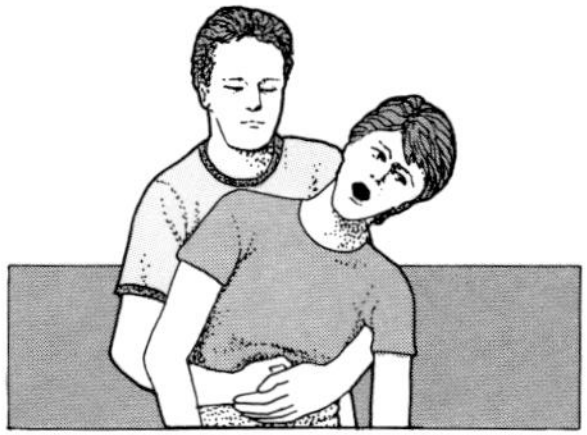

If victim is conscious
Stand behind him with your arms around his waist. Place fist above his navel. With fist of other hand, press into abdomen with four or five upward movements.

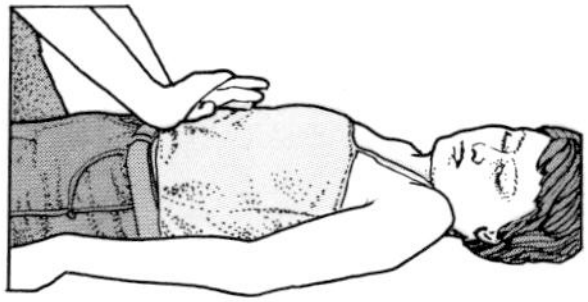

If victim is unconscious
Place him on his back and kneel to one side. Place heel of hand on lower half of victim's chest with other hand on top. Lean forward and with four quick downward thrusts – compress victim's chest.

Electrocution

Electrocution

If the casualty is still in contact with the source of electricity, contact must be broken, or the power removed, immediately. Do not touch the casualty while in contact with electricify, you will risk electrocution yourself.

Treatment for electrocution

Switch off power, or pull out plug, or knock casualty clear of contact with a *dry* lever (wood, newspaper, etc. but not metal). When doing this you must be standing on a dry surface. Do not hold casualty under the armpits, they are likely to be damp. Check if the casualty is breathing. If necessary, clear the airway and give artificial respiration (p. 13) for a prolonged period. When breathing is regular, put in the recovery position (p. 13). Once the casualty is clear of the source of electricity, and breathing has been established, burns, if they have occurred, must be cooled by immersion in cool water or by the application of slowly running water. Get the casualty to hospital quickly.

ACTION IN CASE OF ELECTROCUTION

1 If possible, that is, without risk to yourself, turn off the power at source – or disconnect the power supply.

2 If it is not possible to turn off the power, disconnect the supply by pulling away the cable – but handle only the insulated part of the cable.

3 If all else fails, knock the electrical contact away from the casualty, or knock the casualty away from the contact. Use only a dry non-conductor for this.

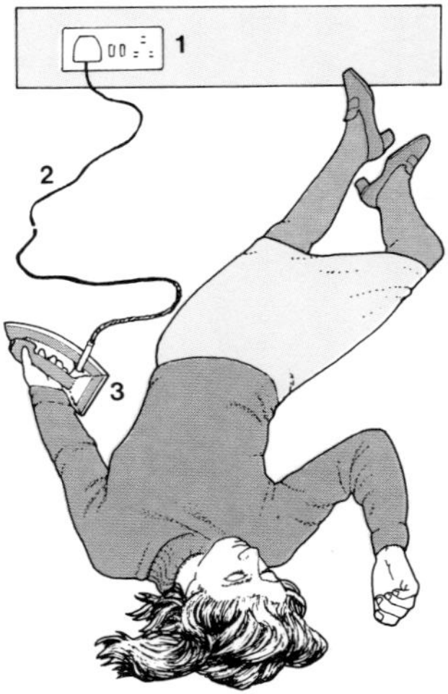

Gassing/Suffocation/Smothering

Gassing	Most households now use natural gas, which is not poisonous. But gassing can still occur from faulty stoves, motor exhaust fumes, etc.
Treatment for gassing	Turn off the source of gas. Remove the casualty to fresh air. Clear the airway, and if not breathing, give artificial respiration (p. 13). When breathing is regular, put in the recovery position (p. 13).
Suffocation	Suffocation occurs when air cannot pass in and out of the lungs. Most cases of suffocation are caused by smoke.
Treatment for suffocation	Remove the casualty from smoke area. Clear the airway, and give artificial respiration (p. 13).
Smothering	Smothering occurs when air cannot reach the mouth or nose.
Treatment for smothering	Remove the obstruction, clear the airway and give artificial respiration (p. 13). When breathing is regular, put in the recovery position (p. 13).

ACTION IN GAS OR SMOKE FILLED ROOMS

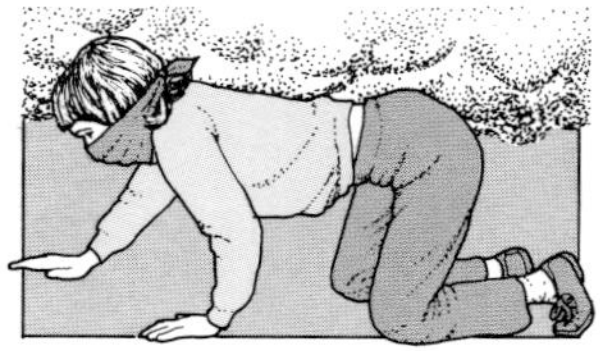

Searching smoke filled areas
Make a face mask with wet cloth, and bend low, or crawl. There is more oxygen at low level.

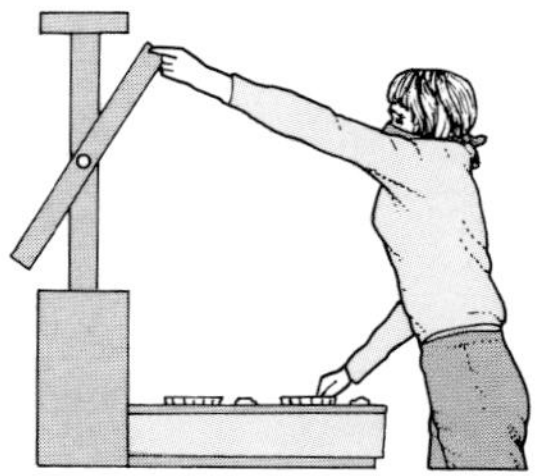

Escaping gas
If possible, turn off the gas supply and then ventilate the room. Do not use naked flames or turn on light.

Remove casualty to fresh air if possible

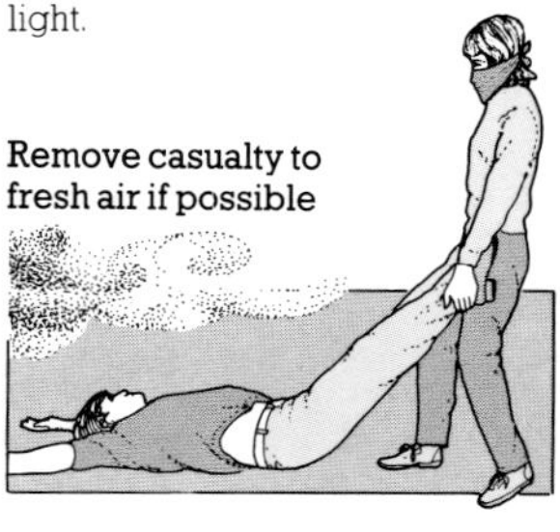

Gassing/Suffocation/Smothering

Asphyxiation general

Collectively, drowning, suffocation by smoke and smothering of young children account for a great many accidental deaths each year. Deep water is not essential to drowning – all that is required to drown is sufficient fluid to block the airway. Most fire victims are not burned, they are suffocated by smoke. Parents seem unaware of the ease with which very young children can suffocate. Clearly, vigilance and preventive measures are of primary importance, but it is also vital to be well practised in the techniques of first aid. In the case of asphyxiation this almost always means the techniques of artificial respiration. In theory, artificial respiration is quite simple – you blow air into the casualty's lungs in order to restart breathing. In practise, it is something which is done best if properly learned. Anyone can do it, and no-one should be deterred if they have not done it before – but it is best to be prepared.

See page 13

THOSE IN DANGER
Babies and young children are particularly prone to smothering by plastic materials.

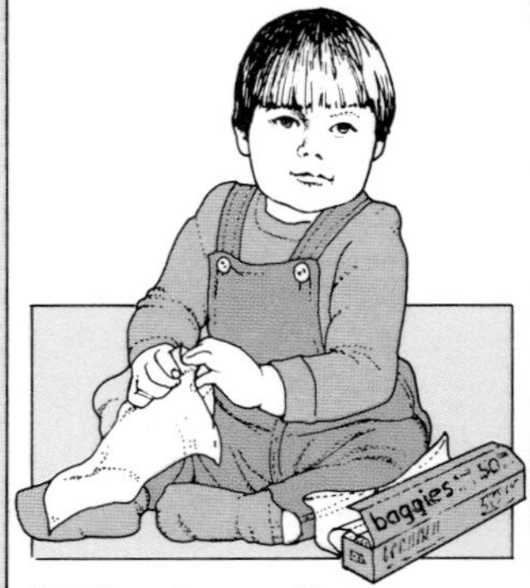

Polythene bags and liners
Keep these, and similar materials away from young children. Plastic bags are very tempting playthings but, if they make contact with the face, they immediately cling and cut off air completely. This rapidly induces panic in children.

Plastic and rubber sheets
Avoid non-porous plastic and rubber sheeting in cots and prams. Babies can become entangled in these materials or fall asleep face down – in either case the plastic may cling and cut off the baby's air supply.

Bleeding

Bleeding is the escape of blood from the vessels which carry it around the body. In *external* bleeding, blood flows from wounds in the skin. *Internal* bleeding is more complicated. Blood may remain inside the body or may be passed from it, i.e. from the lungs or stomach, but wounds will not be visible. Loss of blood from the circulation must be stopped as soon as possible.

A healthy adult has about 6 litres (10 pints) of blood in his circulation. Small amounts can be lost without danger but a loss of 1.2 litres (2 pints) or more (and a much smaller amount in children) can have serious effects on the body.

When blood stops flowing, it will clot and block the damaged vessel. Therefore treatment for severe bleeding aims to: (**a**) stop further loss of blood and weakening of the casualty, (**b**) help blood clotting by resting the casualty, (**c**) get the casualty to hospital quickly for blood replacement.

It will be necessary when treating bleeding, particularly in severe cases, to know how to take the pulse rate and record it. The pulse itself is an important indication of the casualty's condition and should be taken regularly – even after giving first aid.

THE PULSE

A pulse is a throb felt in an artery, corresponding to each heart beat. The throb is caused by an expansion of the artery as the heart beat forces blood along it.

In many injuries, the pulse is a vital indicator of the casualty's condition.

Although the first aider may not know what every change in the strength or rate of the pulse means, it is essential to record such changes so that the hospital can be informed.

NORMAL PULSE RATES	
Adults	60-80 times per minute
Children	90-100 times per minute
Babies	100-140 times per minute

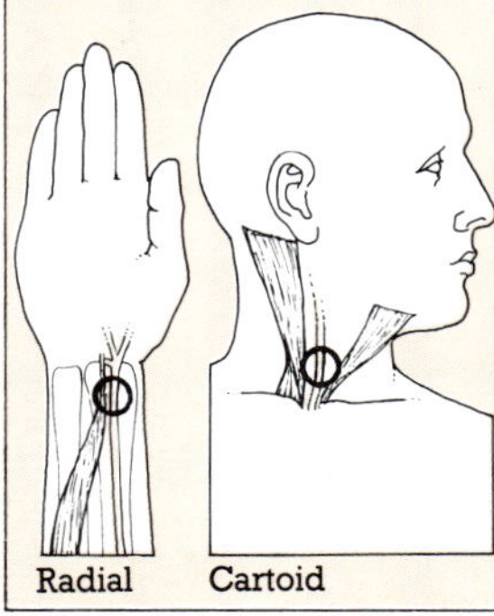

Locating the pulse
The pulse is best found on the under side of the thumb side of the wrist (the *radial* pulse), and the side of the neck below the jaw *(cartoid)*. The cartoid pulse is often the easier to locate – a point worth remembering when speed is essential.

External bleeding

External bleeding Bleeding from an open wound has to be stopped quickly, and the wound covered to prevent infection. When a casualty has severe wounds, he should be treated before being moved, unless there is danger to life in staying put.

Treatment for external bleeding Lay the casualty down, because he may feel faint, and give reassurance. Put direct pressure on the wound with the fingers, using a dressing if one is available. Apply pressure for up to 15 minutes. If the wound is large or gaping, pinch the sides together for 2 minutes before applying pressure. Place a sterile dressing firmly on the wound, cover with a pad of soft material and bandage firmly in position. *Keep everything as clean as possible.* If bleeding re-starts after dressing the wound, do not remove the dressing but add more on top.

A casualty with severe wounds must be removed to hospital as soon as possible.

TAKING THE PULSE

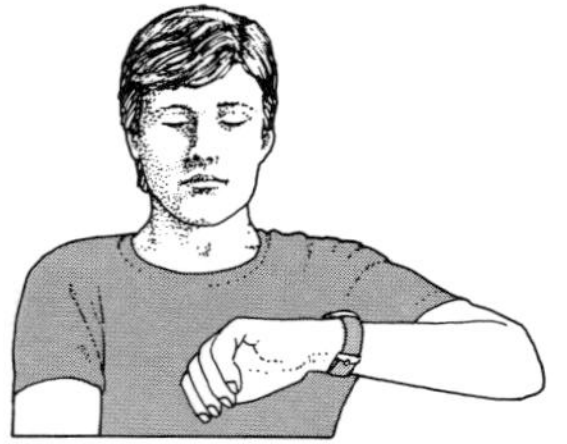

Timing pulse beat
Using a watch with a second hand, count the pulse for 30 seconds and multiply the result by 2.

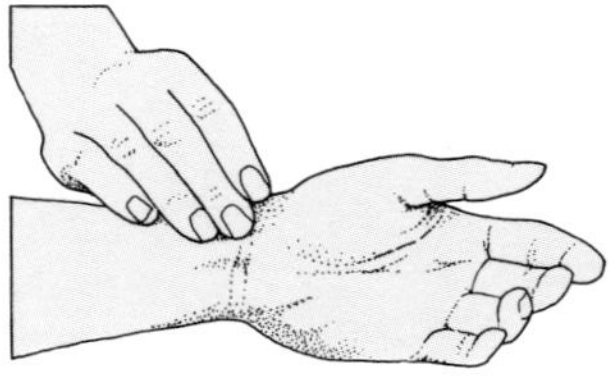

Taking radial pulse
Put 2 or 3 finger tips on the thumb side of the wrist and press lightly.

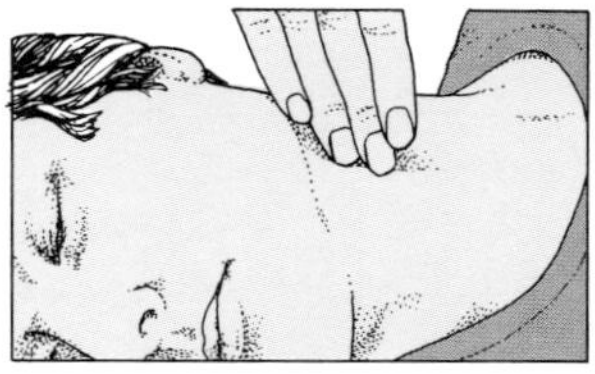

Taking cartoid pulse
Place your finger tips on the side of the neck; do not press too hard.

External bleeding

Foreign body in wound	If a foreign body is embedded in the wound (gravel, metal, pieces of bone), do not attempt to remove it. Instead, put dressings around the wound and pressure to the edge of the wound. Cover and bandage lightly.
Deep wounds	Pack with large sterile dressings up to the surface, then bandage.
Amputated limb	Cover with very firm pad on stump, and apply pressure when bandaging. Raise limb. Keep the torn-off limb, if possible, and transport it to hospital in a polythene bag.
Leg and arm wounds	If a leg is bleeding and a broken bone is not suspected, raise the leg on a chair. If an arm is affected, put in a sling.
General	Examine the casualty for further wounds, especially underneath him, and watch his general condition, in case more padding is required. Note the pulse rate every 5 minutes.

TYPES OF WOUND

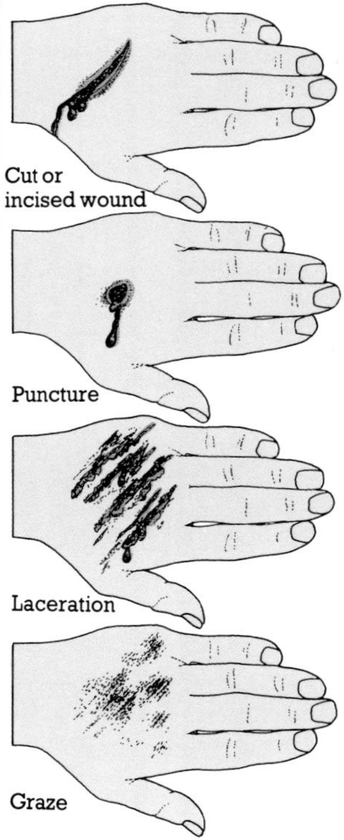

Flesh wounds

Clean cuts may require stitching but usually heal well. Puncture wounds can be deep and there is a danger of infection. Lacerations can be slow to heal, but grazes should heal quickly.

Internal bleeding

Internal bleeding	Bleeding can take place inside the body, often without any visible signs. In this way as much as 2.4 litres (4 pints) of blood can escape and drain into body cavities. It cannot be stopped by pressure, as in external bleeding, but it is important to recognize the signs of internal bleeding, rest the casualty and get him to hospital quickly. Internal bleeding can follow a blow on the body, bullet wounds or broken bones, causing injury to large blood vessels.
Visible signs of bleeding	There may be some visible signs, such as: coughing or vomiting of blood (chest injury; blood discharge from ear, nose or mouth; blood passed in stools or urine; bruising (i.e. bleeding into body tissues).
General condition of casualty	Cold, clammy skin and pallor (more difficult to note in coloured skins). Fast, shallow breathing. Increasing, feeble pulse rate. The casualty complains of faintness, thirst, and is restless and anxious.

ACTION IN CASES OF SEVERE BLEEDING

The chief aims in treating severe bleeding are:

- To stop the flow of blood as soon as possible.
- Prevent further weakening of the casualty.

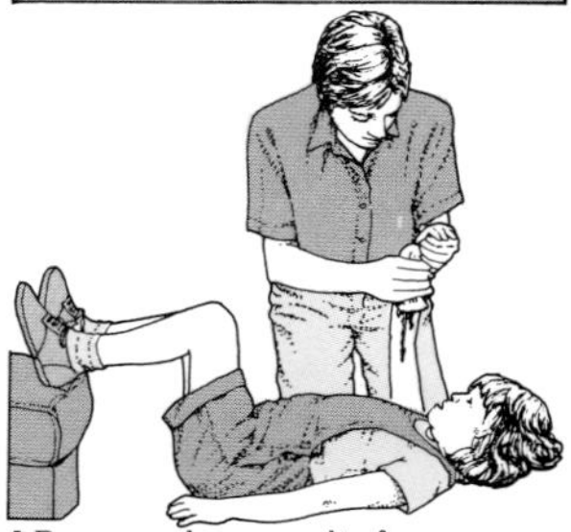

1 Remove the casualty from further danger, if necessary.
2 Lay the casualty down in a comfortable position, preferably with feet higher than head.
3 Apply pressure on the bleeding point or press the sides of the wound together and keep this up for 10-15 minutes. Apply pressure through a dressing if one is available.
4 When the bleeding has stopped, place a dressing over the wound and bandage firmly.
5 Call for medical assistance.

Internal bleeding

Treatment of internal bleeding

Reassure casualty. Get him to rest in the most comfortable position, with head slightly lower than body. If unconscious, put in the recovery position (p. 13). Give nothing by mouth.

If the casualty is lying on the ground put a blanket underneath him. If another blanket is available you may cover him with it, but never put more than one blanket on top of a casualty.

Get to hospital quickly and record pulse rate every 5 minutes.

A casualty with chest injuries must be sent to hospital in a sitting position (*see treatment for fracture of chest page 61*).

ACTION IF INTERNAL BLEEDING SUSPECTED

It internal bleeding is suspected, reassure the casualty and put him in the most comfortable position. Send for medical help or get the casualty to hospital.

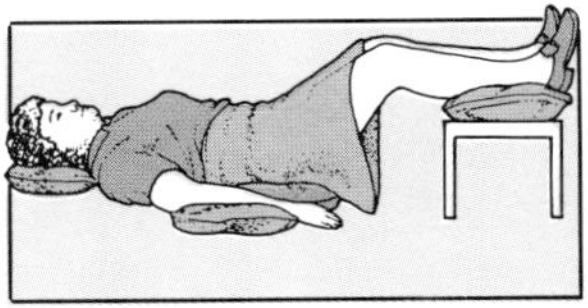

If casualty is conscious
Put into the most comfortable position, preferably with head slightly lower than body.

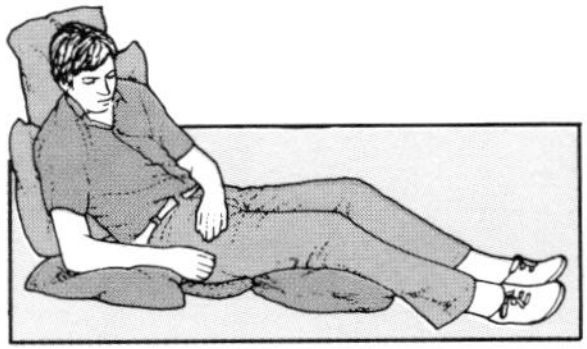

If a chest injury is suspected
Put the casualty into a sitting position and keep him in this position while taking to hospital.

If casualty is unconscious
Put into the recovery position.
See page 13

Unconsciousness

A person who cannot be aroused is deemed to be unconscious, and one must assume that the casualty's brain is not working normally. Immediate treatment is vital.

Common causes of unconsciousness include poisoning, diabetes, asphyxiation, electrocution, epilepsy, fainting, head injuries, heart attacks, severe bleeding and strokes.

General treatment

Check first to see that the casualty is breathing regularly. If not, clear the airway and give artificial respiration (p. 13). Loosen clothing at neck and waist. See that fresh air is available. When breathing is regular, make sure that the airway remains clear. Place the casualty in the recovery position (p. 13), keeping the head slightly lower than body. Check for other injuries, treating them if necessary and get the casualty to hospital. Anyone who has been unconscious, even for a short time, must be seen by a doctor.

While waiting for the ambulance cover the casualty with one blanket only. *Do not give a head pillow.* If the casualty is lying on the ground, put a blanket under him. Record the pulse rate and note any changes in the casualty's condition. Never attempt to give anything by mouth. Do not attempt to rouse and do not leave unattended.

Check for a Medic-alert bracelet or treatment card, indicating medical condition.

If the casualty's breath smells of alcohol, do not assume a case of alcohol poisoning. Casualty may simply have had a drink because of feeling unwell.

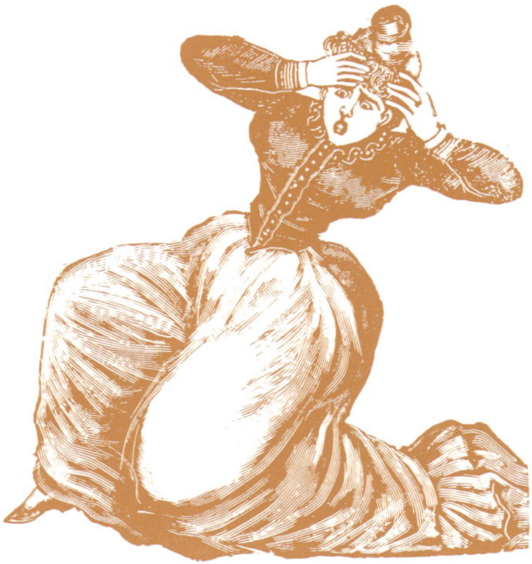

Diabetes

Diabetes

Diabetes is a medical condition in which unconsciousness results from too little or too much insulin in the body. Insulin is a substance manufactured by the body and controls the level of sugar solution in the blood. If too little is produced, extra insulin has to be given. But even when this additional amount is given, unconsciousness can occur if the diabetic person misses a meal, has had too much exercise or an incorrect dose. Known sufferers often carry a treatment card indicating their condition.

Treatment of diabetes

A known, or suspected, diabetic who feels unwell should be given a sweetened drink or lumps of sugar. Failure to provide this simple treatment may result in unconsciousness. If the casualty is discovered in an unconscious state, or becomes unconscious, give nothing by mouth.
Put in the recovery position (p. 13); keep the airway clear; do not leave unattended and get the casualty to hospital.

ACTION IN CASE OF UNCONSCIOUSNESS
If a casualty has been unconscious, even for a short time, he must be seen by a doctor. Immediate treatment is vital – unconsciousness may lead quickly to death.

- Move the casualty away from further damage.
- Check to see if the casualty is breathing regularly. If not, clear the airway and give artificial respiration *(see pages 12-13).* Make sure that the airway remains clear after breathing has recommenced.
- Place the casualty in the recovery position, with head slightly lower than body.
- Check for, and treat, any other injuries.
- Get the casualty to hospital.

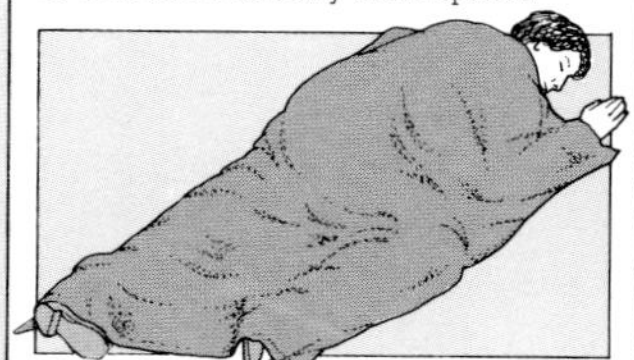

While waiting for ambulance
Cover the casualty with one blanket, but do not give a pillow. Do not attempt to rouse or give anything by mouth.

Epilepsy

Epilepsy

Epilepsy is a condition in which the sufferer has convulsive attacks. Any age can be affected and it varies from mild attacks (often with no loss of consciousness) to major attacks with abrupt loss of consciousness. Sufferers often carry a Medic-alert bracelet or an SOS Talisman.

Signs of major attack

The casualty suddenly becomes unconscious and falls to ground. Body becomes rigid and goes into convulsions with limbs jerking. Breathing is noisy, and there may be frothing at the mouth. Sometimes there will be loss of control of bladder and bowels. An attack may last a few seconds or several minutes, then the jerking stops, the casualty relaxes and passes into deep sleep. When recovering, he can be dazed and exhausted. Often, when recovering consciousness, the casualty will behave as if he does not know what he is doing. This condition is called post-epileptic automatism.

MEDIC ALERT
A casualty may be carrying a medic-alert card or bracelet indicating a condition such as diabetes or epilepsy. Do not forget to look for one of these.

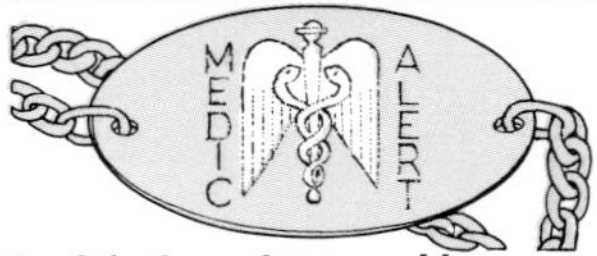

Look for bracelet or necklace

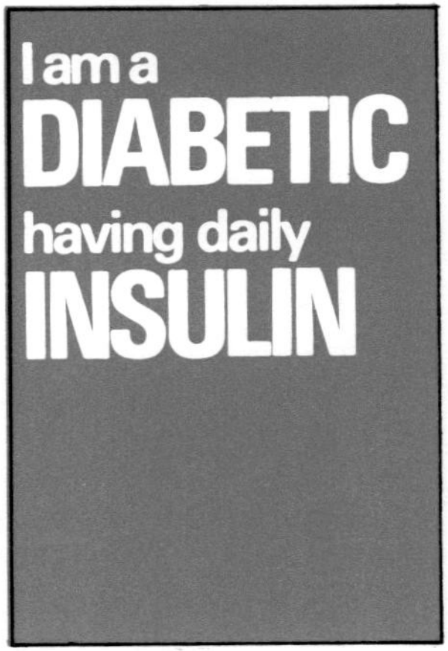

Look for a card
A medic-alert card will give you the probable reason for unconsciousness.

Epilepsy

Treatment of epilepsy

Remain calm, and move casualty only if there is danger from traffic, fire, nearness of furniture etc. Let the attack run its course and do not try to stop the jerking or restrain the casualty in any way. *Do not put anything between the casualty's teeth.* Do not give anything by mouth. Loosen any tight clothing. When convulsions stop, turn the casualty into the recovery position (p. 13) and stay with him until a normal state returns. Reassure him.
Although the attack causes loss of consciousness, the casualty should recover without medical aid. But if injury has occurred during the fall, or the casualty has a series of fits without regaining consciousness, then a doctor or ambulance must be called.

Minor epileptic attacks

Many sufferers from epilepsy seldom experience a major attack, but may have recurring minor attacks. Fixed, staring eyes and a pale skin may be the first, and sometimes the only, signs of an attack.

BRAIN CONCUSSION
A disturbance of the working of the brain, caused by a blow or 'shaking'.

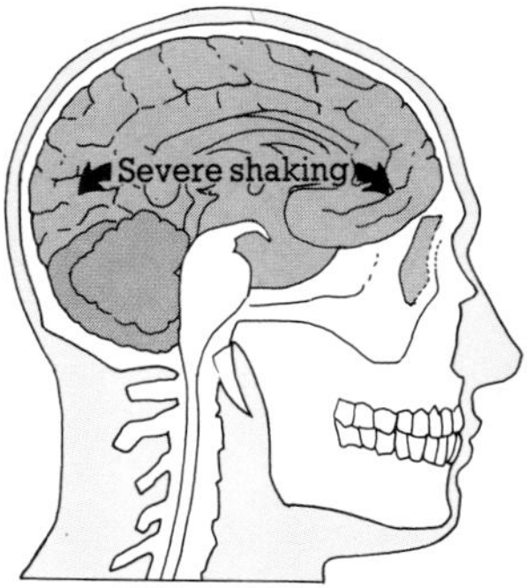

SIGNS OF CONCUSSION

- Possible unconsciousness
- Shallow breathing
- Pale, cold, clammy skin
- Nausea during recovery
- Dazed after recovering consciousness
- Loss of memory
- Heacache

Any casualty who suffers unconsciousness, even for a short period, must see a doctor. Concussion may not seem serious, but it is a brain injury.

Concussion/Compression

Head injuries	Scalp wounds, or fractures to the skull bone may be present, with or without brain injury. But if any period of unconsciousness follows head injury, the casualty must see a doctor.
Concussion	Concussion is a temporary breakdown in the normal working of the brain, following a severe "shaking-up" of the brain inside the skull. Usually the casualty recovers completely within a few days.
Signs of concussion	Unconsciousness, usually for a short time. Shallow breathing; pale, cold and clammy skin. When casualty recovers he is dazed, and may vomit, have a headache and remember nothing before or after the injury.
Compression of brain	If unconsciousness continues, compression of brain may be present. This is due to pressure on the brain, either from fragments of broken bone, or from an escape of blood from damaged blood vessels.

BRAIN COMPRESSION
Pressure on the brain, caused by fluid or blood, or by a depressed fracture of the skull.

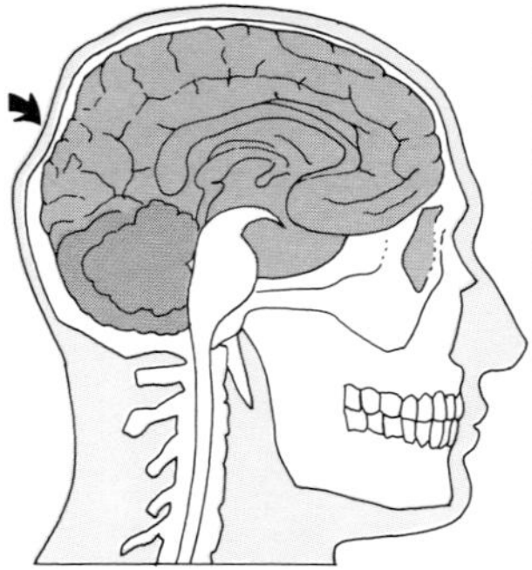

SIGNS OF COMPRESSION

- Unconsciousness, sometimes following a period of stupor
- Twitching of limbs
- Convulsions
- Slow pulse
- Noisy breathing
- Raised temperature
- Dilated or unequal pupils in the eyes

- A casualty who becomes unconscious after a blow on the head must see a doctor as soon as possible.

Concussion/Compression

Signs of compression of the brain	Headaches, drowsiness, then unconsciousness. In the early stages there may be twitching and convulsions. A slowing pulse, noisy breathing and raised body temperature. There may be some weakness or paralysis on one side of the body. The pupils of the eyes may be dilated and may not react to light.
Treatment for concussion and compression	Watch breathing, keep the airway clear, give artificial respiration if needed. When breathing regularly, put in the recovery position, with head slightly lowered (p. 13). Get a doctor or ambulance urgently.
Concussion and compression *general*	Both of these conditions may not be revealed until some time after an accident or a blow on the head. Neither is necessarily preceded, or accompanied by, unconsciousness. Compression, which is often caused by blood or fluid inside the skull, can take several hours to become apparent. Any casualty with symptoms must see a doctor.

SERIOUS HEAD INJURY
Abnormal appearance of the pupils of the eye can indicate a serious head injury.

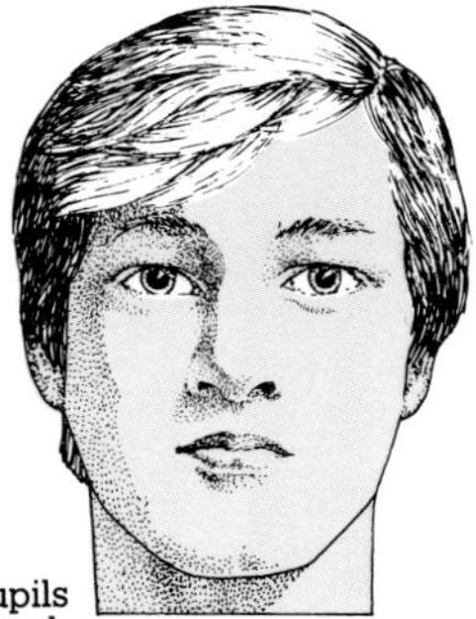

Pupils very large

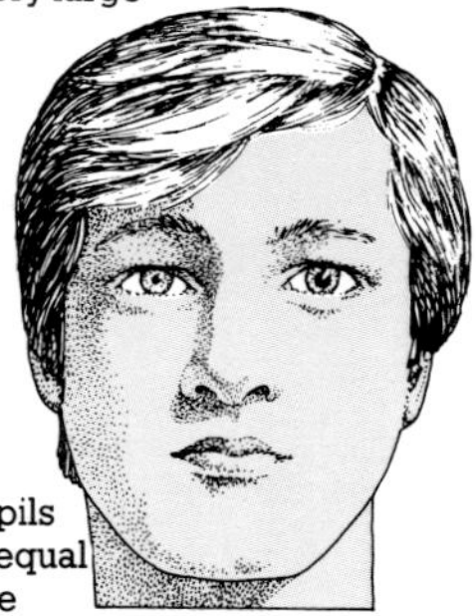

Pupils unequal size

A quick test
By shining a torch or other light into the casualty's eyes you can quickly check normal responses or abnormal signs.

Heart attack

Heart attack

A heart attack occurs when the blood supply to the heart muscle is reduced. It is most likely to take place in middle-aged or elderly people, especially those who smoke, have little exercise and are overweight.

Signs of heart attack

Sudden onset of pain in chest, often described as a 'tight band'. The pain may also extend along the arms. Irregular, feeble pulse. Pale, clammy skin. Shortness of breath. Possibly unconsciousness.

Treatment for heart attack

Send for ambulance, and keep the casualty resting quietly in most comfortable position, usually semi-recumbent. Loosen any tight clothing. Tell the casualty to breathe deeply. Do not give anything by mouth. If breathing fails, see that the airway is clear and give artificial respiration (p.13). Record the pulse rate every 5 minutes. If breathing is regular but the casualty is unconscious, put in the recovery position (p. 13) and get to hospital quickly.

SIGNS OF A HEART ATTACK

- Severe chest pain
- Pain moves into arms
- Irregular or feeble pulse
- Pale and clammy skin
- Breathlessness

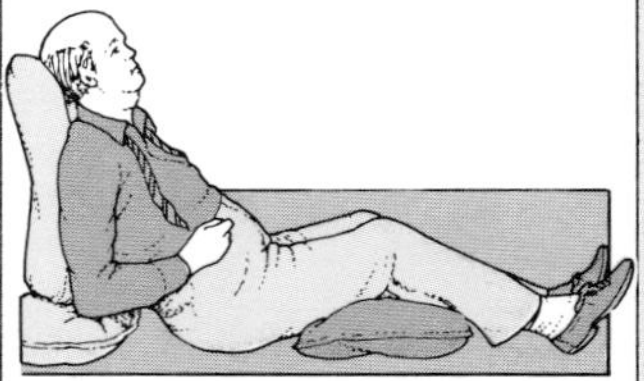

Recovery positions
If the casualty is conscious, he should rest in a half sitting position – supported by cushions. If unconscious, he should be put into the recovery position *(see page 13)*

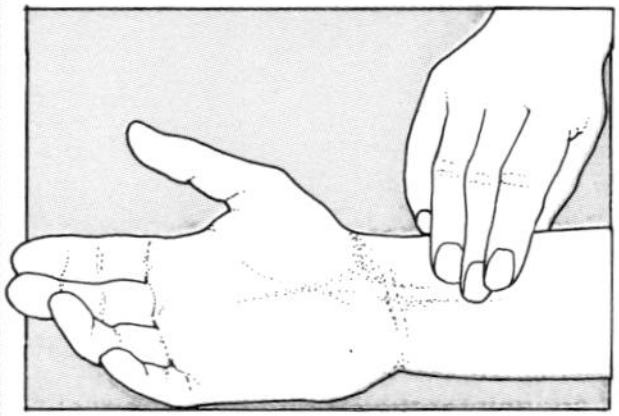

Pulse rate
Check the casualty's pulse rate every five minutes while waiting for the ambulance. Report changes to the hospital.
See page 39 for pulse rate

Stroke

Stroke (apoplexy)	A stroke is the term used to describe damage in the brain from bleeding due to a burst blood vessel in the brain, or from blockage of a blood vessel. In severe cases it can cause loss of consciousness and paralysis down one side of the body. If a small blood vessel is involved, there can be a complete recovery.
Those affected	The middle-aged to elderly, those suffering from high blood pressure and (rarely) young people with weakness of blood vessel wall since birth.
Signs of a stroke	Sudden collapse, often without warning but sometimes following a headache. Noisy breathing, possible frothing at nose and mouth, pallor and rapid, strong pulse.
Treatment for a stroke	Clear the airway, put in the recovery position (p. 13). Loosen any tight clothing, and do not leave the casualty unattended. Get to hospital.

SIGNS OF A STROKE

- Sudden collapse
- Noisy breathing
- Frothing at nose/mouth
- Rapid, strong pulse
- Limpness on one side

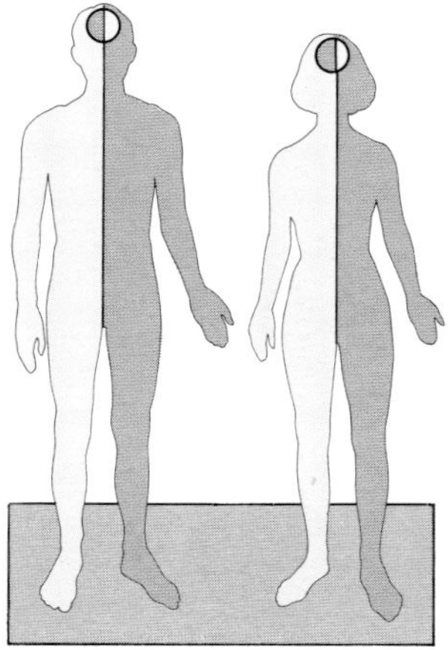

What is a stroke?
A stroke is what occurs when the blood supply to part of the brain is impaired. The part of the brain not receiving its proper supply of blood ceases to work. The right side of the brain controls the left side of the body and vice versa, so the effect on the body will be on the side opposite to the damage in the brain.

PROCEDURE IN CASE OF ROAD ACCIDENTS

- **Warn oncoming traffic**
  Put out a red reflecting signal 45m (50yds) before the obstruction (140m/150yds on highways) on the same side of the road. If you have no warning devices, get a helper to flag down traffic.
- **Protect survivors and helpers**
  Switch off the engines of all vehicles involved; apply handbrakes or use wheel chocks. Put out any fires with fire extinguishers, blankets, etc. Keep clear of leaking gas tanks, chemicals, etc.
- **Get message to emergency services**
  Give the exact site of the accident; the number of victims; number of vehicles involved and their type; number of victims trapped; whether fire is involved, and the services required.
- **Do not smoke**
  Or let others do so.
- **Give First Aid to those most in need**
  Minor injuries can wait for treatment.

Remember ABC – Airways, Breathing, Circulation.

- **Are the airways clear?**
  Is the victim breathing? Give artificial respiration if needed.
- **Is the victim bleeding?**
  Stop bleeding by pressure and cover wounds.
- **Is the victim unconscious?**
  If breathing is regular, try to move into the recovery position.
- **Treat any serious injuries.**
- **Report all action taken to emergency services**
- **Do not make matters worse**
  By moving injured victims before the emergency services arrive (unless there is danger from fire).

GENERAL FIRST AID

If the casualty is breathing normally, and first aid has been given for any severe bleeding and unconsciousness, then other serious injuries must be treated.

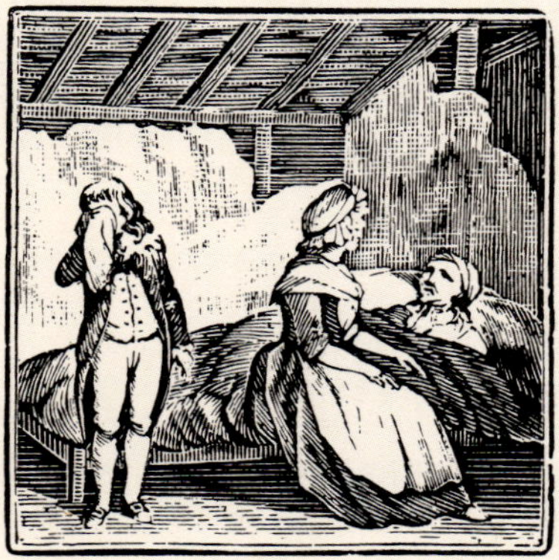

Burns & scalds

Burns and scalds
general

Burns are injuries to the body tissues caused by dry heat: fire, friction, electricity. Scalds are burns caused by moist heat: steam, hot liquids, hot fats. Chemical burns are caused by corrosive liquids.

All burns cause great pain and shock.

Burning of the skin can cause reddening, blister formation, and in serious burns, tissue destruction. Burns are either *superficial* or *deep*, depending on the depth of damage to tissues. Large areas of burning, even superficial, will result in serious fluid loss.

All burned tissue retains heat and will do further damage unless cooled quickly. The cooling will relieve pain and by preventing further tissue destruction may lessen the treatment required in hospital.

Remember that most accidents which result in burns occur in the home and could have been prevented with adequate fire precautions.

ACTION IN CASE OF BURNS AND SCALDS

- Remove cause from casualty or vice versa
- Cool burned area quickly
- Apply a sterile, dry dressing
- Replace fluid loss by giving small quantities of water
- Seek medical advice

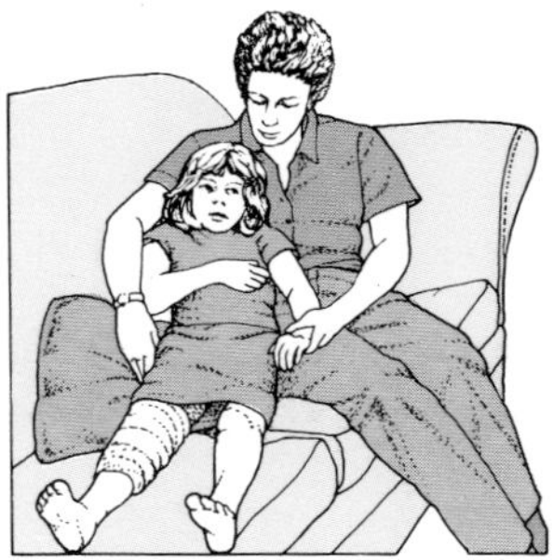

Reassure and comfort casualty
Once emergency treatment has been administered, it is necessary to give the casualty plenty of comfort and reassurance. A combination of shock and severe pain is usually present in cases of burns and scalds – especially where children are affected.

Burns & scalds

Treatment for burns

Prompt first aid for burns will not only save life but may also prevent permanent damage.
If the casualty's clothing is on fire, smother flames in a rug or coat, or dowse with water, taking care not to burn yourself. Make the casualty lie down – standing or going into open air could spread the fire. Reassure the casualty. Treat the largest burned area first. *(See page 25.)*

Cooling burns

Cool burned area by soaking (or flooding) with cold water for at least 15 minutes. Use a bucket, sink, or gently running tap. Cooling is essential.
If the face is burned, use a cold compress, but do not rub the burned area. When the area is cooled, cover with sterile, dry dressings and bandage lightly. Dressings should be larger than the burned area. Cotton sheeting may be used for bandaging. For a burned face, cover with a gauze mask – cut a hole for breathing. Always bandage over burned clothing. Remove any tight-fitting

DEGREES OF BURN
Burning of the skin will cause reddening, possibly blistering and, in serious cases, extensive tissue destruction. Burns may be deep or superficial, depending on the area of the burn.

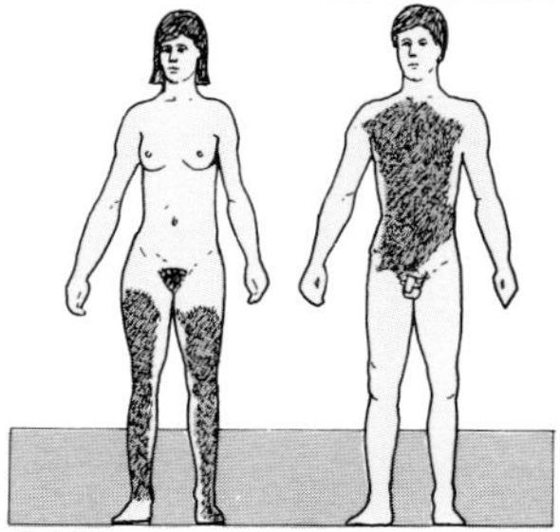

Adults
Anyone receiving burns to the equivalent of the shaded area requires hospital treatment

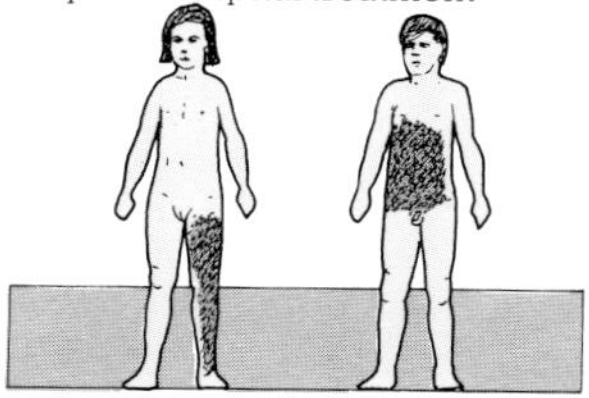

Children
Children require hospital treatment with a smaller area of burns than adults.

Burns & scalds

Cooling burns *continued*

articles, such as shoes, rings on fingers etc. Then, put casualty in a comfortable position (burned leg on a cushion, arm in a sling) and get to hospital quickly.
When body tissue is burnt, body fluids are lost and need replacement. If the casualty is conscious, give about half a cupful of water by mouth every 10-15 minutes until he reaches hospital.

Treatment for scalds

Reassure the casualty.
Immediately soak affected part in cold water. Remove wet clothes if they are not stuck to body. Treat as for burns (above).

Scalded mouth

Scalded mouths usually result from drinking hot liquids, or when a child puts a kettle spout in the mouth. Scalding will cause swelling and difficulty in breathing. If scalding is severe, put the casualty in the recovery position (p. 13). If breathing stops, give artificial respiration (p. 13). When the casualty is conscious, give him ice cubes to suck and get to hospital.

TREATMENT FOR BURNS AND SCALDS

- Cool burned area
- Dress the burn
- Make casualty comfortable
- Reassure, and give drinks

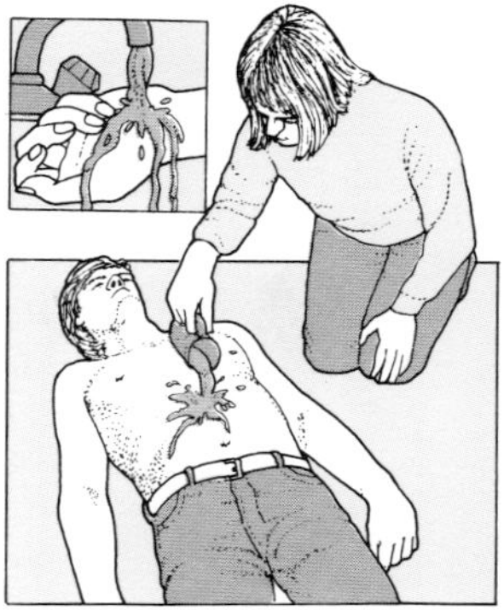

Reduce heat
The importance of cooling burned areas cannot be overemphasised. Without cooling treatment, heat will remain in the burned area for several minutes and will cause further tissue destruction. The burned, or scalded, part should be soaked in cold water for at least 10 minutes after the accident. Gently running water provides the most effective treatment. If you cannot use a tap, use a watering can or a soaked sponge.

Burns & scalds

Treatment for chemical burns	Wash the affected area very thoroughly to rinse off the chemical and prevent further damage. Use running water for 10-15 minutes. Remove affected clothing and soak in water. Do not contaminate yourself. Treat as for burns (above) and get to hospital quickly.
Chemical burns to eye	Chemical burns of the eye can cause great damage, even loss of sight. Get the casualty to lie down and hold his eyelids apart with finger and thumb; pour cold water continuously over front of eye from nose side, so that chemical does not run into the other eye. Continue for 10-15 minutes, while opening and closing the eyelids, until the chemical is washed away. Cover with dressing and get to hospital quickly.
Electrical burns	*See page 35 and above.*
Sunburn	*See page 88*
Friction burns	*See page 76*

DRESSINGS FOR BURNS

Wherever there is tissue damage there is a risk of infection. Burned areas are particularly susceptible and should be covered with dry, sterile dressings. They can be improvised from clean, cotton sheeting or handkerchiefs, but not from cotton wool, lint or other fluffy materials. Dressings should be large enough to cover more than the burned area.

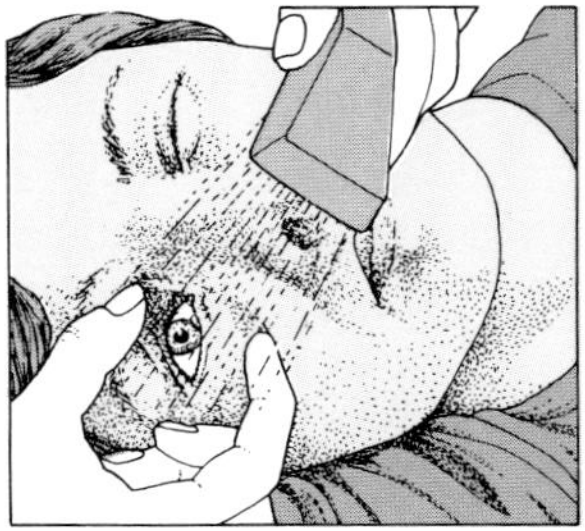

Chemical burn to eye
Get casualty to lie down and, while holding the eyelids open, pour, or spray, cold water across the eye. Do this for several minutes not letting the chemical reach the other eye.

Scalded mouth
Ice cubes will soothe a scalded mouth – but make sure the casualty is fully conscious.

Burned face
A burned face can be cooled with a cold compress.

Fractures

Causes of fracture

Fractures are broken or cracked bones usually caused by direct violence, such as a body blow, or indirect violence, such as the fracture of a collar bone after a fall onto an outstretched hand.

Types of fracture

Closed fractures – when the covering skin is not broken. Open fractures – when there is a wound leading down to the fracture, or when bone ends may stick out of the skin.

Both kinds of fracture can cause damage to internal tissues and organs. Once the wound of an open fracture has been covered, first aid is the same as for any broken bone. Fractures must be confirmed by X-ray examination. Treat a suspected fracture as a fracture.

Immobilizing fractures

Immobilize the injured part by using the body as a splint where possible, i.e., tying an injured leg to the uninjured one. If there is no suspected injury to the lower half of body, raise the legs higher than the head. Cover with one blanket.

SIGNS OF FRACTURE

- **Pain/tenderness** in region of injury. Not always severe, but usually present.
- **Swelling and bruising** are often present.
- **Deformity** may be apparent, especially with broken limbs.
- **Loss of power** in a limb will usually accompany a fracture.
- **Unnatural movement** – a broken limb may move abnormally, or with a grating sensation if the fracture is complicated.
- **Internal bleeding** is often present to some degree.
- **Recent history** – has the casualty been recently injured in any way?

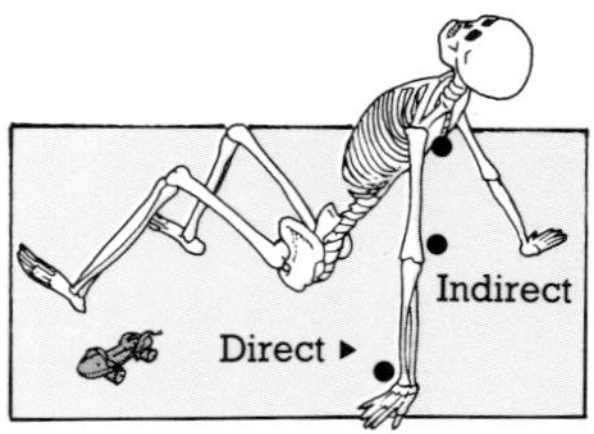

Causes of fracture
Fractures may be caused by *direct* violence, e.g. a broken wrist after a fall onto the hand, or *indirect*, e.g. a broken collar bone from the same fall.

Fractures

Immobilizing fractures *continued*

Give nothing by mouth.
Do not attempt to straighten a limb before immobilizing. If you are using splints, pad well before bandaging. If a limb is injured, immobilize the joints above and below the fracture. Before bandaging, pad the hollows and bony points of that part of the body affected. Use natural hollows such as under the knee or small of the back to pass bandages under, and then slide up or down as required.
If necessary, improvise splints from a walking stick, folded newspaper, etc.
Tie all bandages with reef knots (to prevent them slipping) on the uninjured side.
Do not tie too tightly and watch the circulation in toes and fingers. If they become blue, loosen the bandage slightly. Record pulse rate. Report all such changes to hospital.

Skull and jaw fractures

Fractures of the skull can cause brain damage (*see Head Injuries, p 47*).

TYPES OF FRACTURE

- **Simple fracture**
When a bone is broken cleanly, with no fragmentation.
- **Greenstick fracture**
A bone that is only partially broken – as if bent.
- **Compound fracture**
A bone broken in more than one place.
- **Complicated fracture**
Where the broken bone damages nerves or blood vessels.
- **Open fracture**
Where the broken bone punctures the skin and becomes exposed.

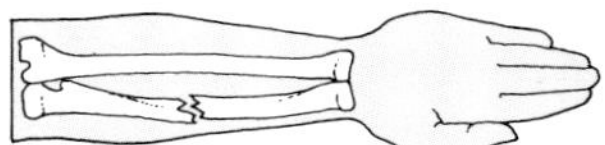
Simple

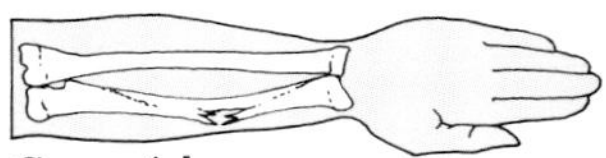
Greenstick

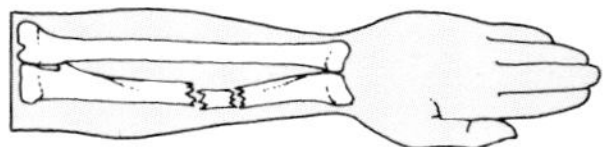
Compound

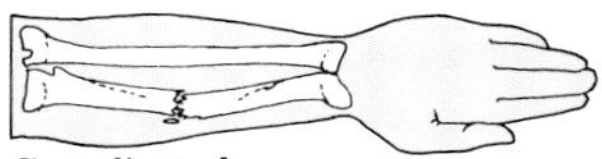
Complicated

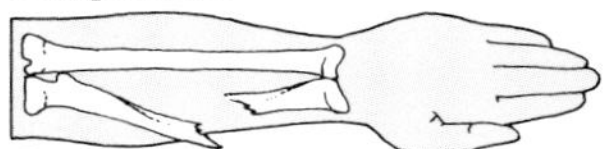
Open

Fractures

Treatment of skull and jaw fractures	Keep airway clear, give artificial respiration if necessary (p. 13). When breathing regularly, put in the recovery position (p. 13). Cover any wound with a dry dressing. If the ear is bleeding, do not plug. Support a broken jaw with bandage and tie on top of head. Keep airway clear. Check pulse rate. Get to hospital quickly: if unconscious, in recovery position, if conscious, in sitting position.
Neck and spine fractures	These are very serious injuries and great care must be taken to prevent further damage. The spine contains the spinal cord, and any injury to this cord can cause permanent paralysis.
Signs of fractured spine	Possible unconsciousness. If conscious, the casualty may complain of pain in the back. There may be numbness or loss of power or sensation in limbs. A known history of injury in the region of the spine should cause the first aider to suspect spinal damage.

IMMOBILIZING FRACTURES

Where possible, use the body as a splint to immobilize fractures of the upper and lower limbs.

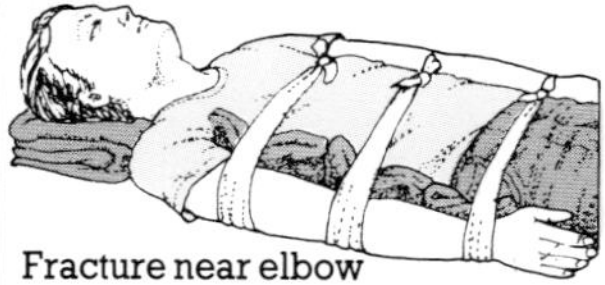

Fracture near elbow

Put padding between the arm and the body and tie the limb to the body with broad bandages: at the wrist and above the site of fracture.

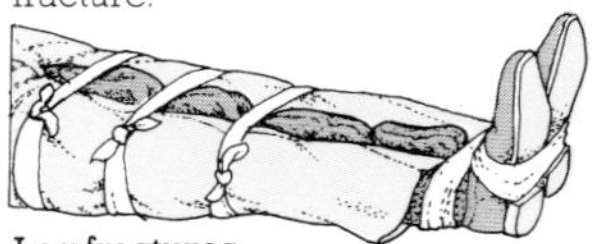

Leg fractures

Put padding in the natural hollows to lessen pain. Take the good leg to the injured one and secure with broad bandages above and below the fracture.

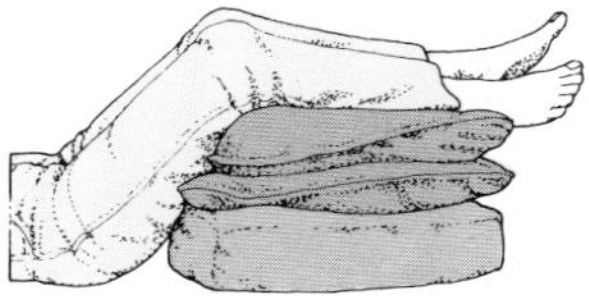

Feet and ankles

Support the feet with cushions or substantial padding.

Fractures

Treatment of spine injury

If a casualty is unconscious, this is the one time when he must not be placed in the recovery position. Watch breathing, keep the airway clear and give artificial respiration (p. 13) if needed. Do not give a head pillow.

If the casualty is conscious, try to find out (without disturbing him) if he can feel pain in his limbs. Even if touch and sensation appear normal treat a suspected back injury very carefully. Do not hurry and do not move the casualty until several helpers are available. Then, if the casualty is lying on the ground, put a blanket under him and keep in the face-upward position. Get to hospital. When the blanket is under the casualty he can then be lifted very carefully, without letting him or the blanket sag, and a stretcher slid under the blanket.

Treatment of neck fracture

Keep the neck well supported with a collar to restrict movement. A temporary collar can be made by folding a newspaper into a stiff band, about 10 cm (4 inches) wide.

USUAL LOCATIONS OF SKULL/FACE/JAW FRACTURES

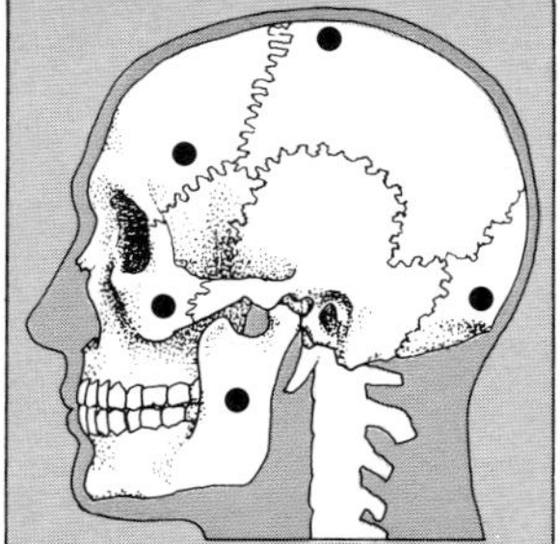

The head is particularly vulnerable to injury. The top and base of the skull, the temple, jaw and cheek bones are most at risk.

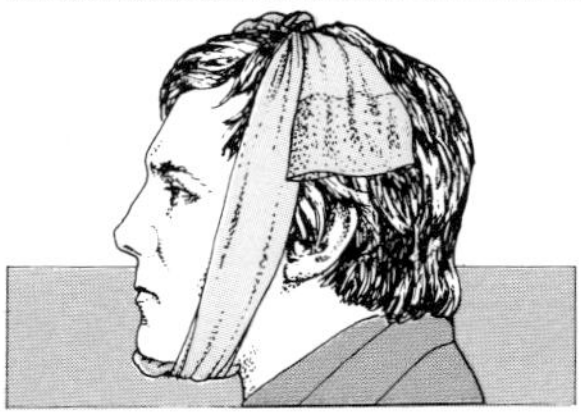

Support for fractured jaw
A fractured jaw is a very painful injury and adequate support must be provided. A bandage can be improvised from a scarf or other fairly soft material. Bring the bandage up from the jaw and tie on top of the head.

Fractures

Chest fracture

The chest is formed by a bony cage of ribs which protect the heart and lungs. If ribs are fractured, there may not be outward signs.

Signs of chest fracture

The casualty complains of pain in the chest, which is worse on coughing or deep breathing. If a rib has pierced a lung, he may cough up frothy blood.

Treatment of chest injury

If a fractured rib is suspected support the arm on injured side in an arm sling (see p. 17).

If it is an open fracture, and a chest wound is present through which air could be 'sucked in', this must be covered at once to keep all air out.

Cover the wound quickly with a sterile dry dressing. Put over the dressing a thick layer of cotton wool or a piece of polythene, large enough to exclude all air. Fix securely in place with a firm bandage or adhesive plaster. Loosen tight clothing; reassure the casualty and record pulse rate.

IMMOBILIZING A NECK FRACTURE

A temporary collar made from newspaper will provide adequate support for the neck.

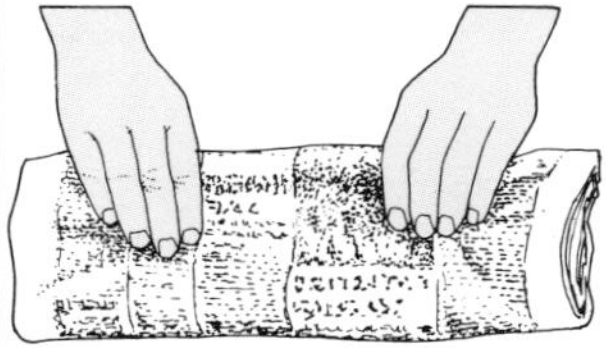

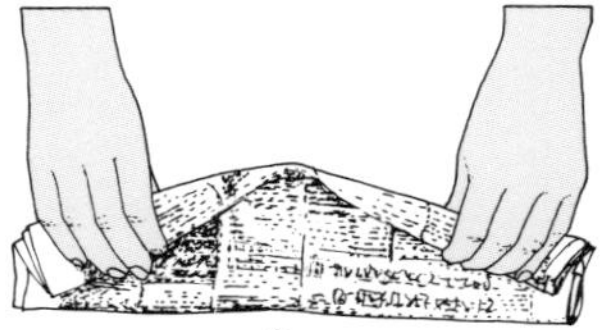

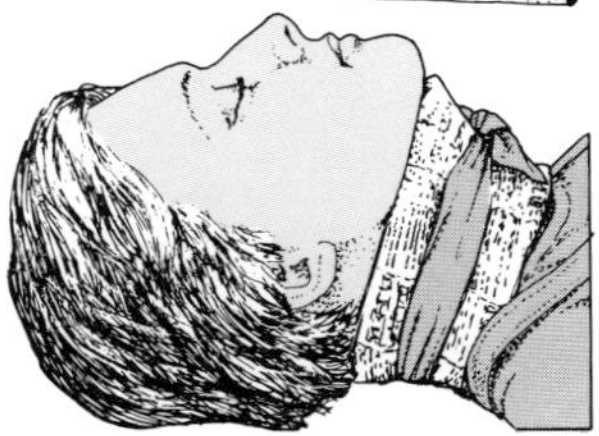

How to improvise a collar

1 Fold a newspaper into a broad band.

2 Turn in the edges to prevent chafing.

3 Wrap the collar completely around the neck and secure with a bandage or necktie.

Fractures

Shoulder and upper arm fractures	Shoulder injuries (invariably to the collar bone) are usually caused by the indirect force of falling onto an outstretched hand. Upper arm fractures may involve the elbow joint.
Treatment of upper arm fractures	Cover any wounds. Place a pad between arm and chest and gently bend the elbow to bring the forearm diagonally across the chest. Support the arm in an arm sling (p. 17). Get to hospital in sitting position.
Elbow fractures	These fractures can be dangerous, particularly in children, because a large artery lies very near the elbow joint. If the arm is bent forcibly, bone fragments could damage the artery.
Treatment of elbow fractures	Take casualty to hospital on a stretcher. If the arm is already bent treat as a fracture of the upper arm (see above). If the arm is straight, do not bend. Bandage firmly to side of the body in the most comfortable position, with padding between arm and body.

PUTTING BLANKET UNDER CASUALTY

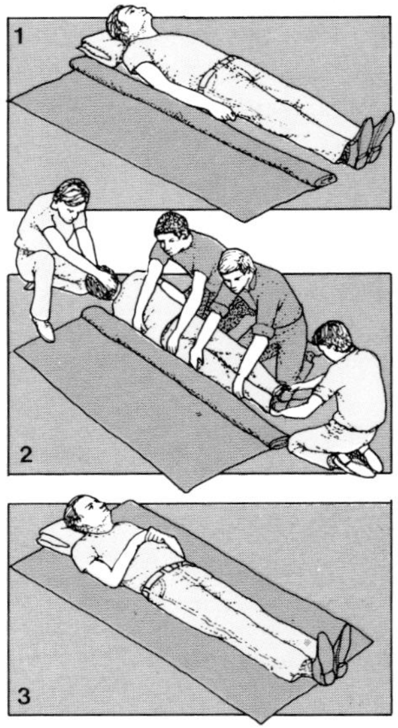

1 Roll the blanket lengthwise for half its width and place beside casualty.
2 Slowly and gently, turn casualty on his side while supporting his feet and head by *gently* pulling them away from his body. Place the blanket roll close to his back.
3 Turn him back over the roll and on to his other side. Roll the blanket out flat and lay him down.
NB *If the casualty has a suspected spine or neck injury, wait until at least four helpers are available.*

Fractures

Lower arm, wrist and hand fractures	Support in an arm sling (p. 17) with the arm straight across the body. Get to hospital in sitting position.
Pelvic fractures	The pelvis is a bone at the lower end of the spine, which supports the lower abdomen. Abdominal organs, including the bladder, lie within the pelvic region, and a complication of this fracture can be damaging to the urinary system.
Signs of pelvic fracture	Pain in hip region, possibly in groins. Standing is painful or impossible. Desire to pass water.
Treatment of pelvic fracture	Lay casualty on his back in the most comfortable position. Tell him to avoid passing water if possible. Knees can be bent slightly, and a folded garment put underneath. *Check for signs of internal bleeding.* Put padding between the knees and ankles, then tie them together. Put a broad bandage around the hips. Get to hospital on a stretcher.

IDENTIFYING A PELVIC FRACTURE

The casualty will have pain in the hip region and, possibly, in the groin. Standing will be painful or impossible. There may be a desire to pass water.

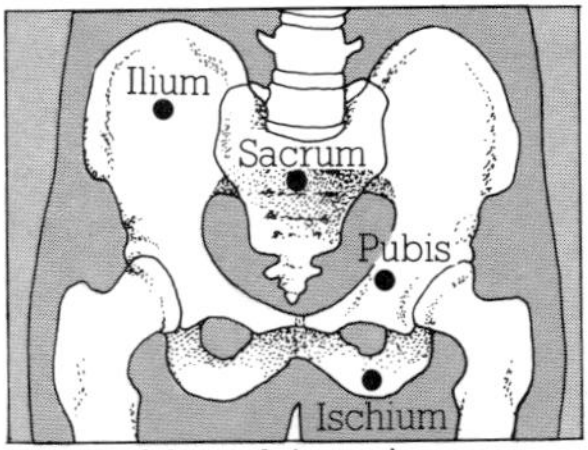

Bones of the pelvic region

IDENTIFYING A CHEST FRACTURE

The casualty will have pain in the chest which may be severe on coughing or deep breathing. If a rib has pierced a lung, he may cough up frothy blood.

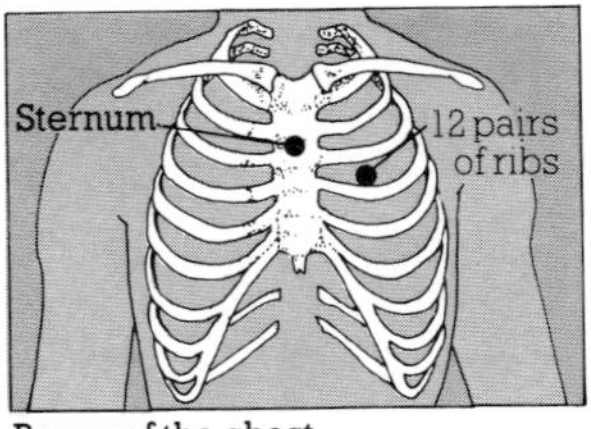

Bones of the chest

Fractures

Leg and foot fractures	Legs are often fractured in accidents, and as large bones are involved, there can be extensive internal bleeding.
Treatment when one leg is injured	Cover any wound with a dry dressing. Do not attempt to push back any protruding bone ends. Use the sound leg as a splint: put pads between thighs, knees and ankles, gradually move sound leg towards injured leg, supporting the feet (*see page 59*). Tie feet, knees and ankles together. Add more bandages above and below the fracture. Get to hospital on a stretcher.
Treatment when both legs are injured	Use splints if available, either to stretch from armpits to feet, or to place between legs. Put pads between thighs, knees and ankles and carefully try to ease each leg to a normal position by pulling slowly and firmly. Never push the limbs towards the body. Put splint(s) in position and tie firmly. If no splint is available, bandage the legs together, putting reef knots on the least injured side.

FOOT FRACTURES
Footwear should be loosened but not removed. Raise the injured foot and place it on some kind of cushioning material. Tie the foot to the cushion and send the casualty to hospital lying down.

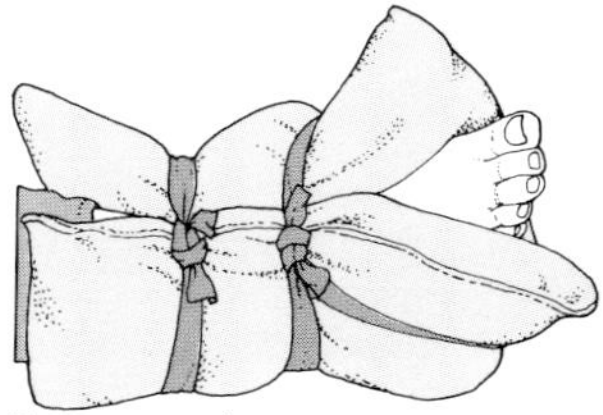

Treatment of foot fracture

When both legs are injured
With pads between the knees, thighs and ankles, gently pull the legs into a normal position. Tie splints (which should stretch from the armpits to the ankles) into position with broad bandages.
See also page 59

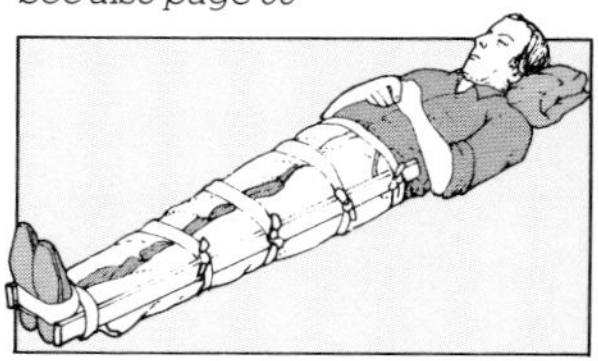

Dislocation

General	Dislocation occurs only in moveable joints, and can be associated with a fracture.
Causes of dislocation	A twist or severe wrench, which displaces the bones from their normal position and tears surrounding ligaments and muscles.
Signs of dislocation	Pain (which can be severe); inability to move joint normally, deformity, swelling and bruising – all similar to fracture symptoms.
Treatment of suspected dislocation	If it is doubtful whether the injury is dislocation or fracture, treat as a fracture. Do not try to put the bones back into normal position. Move the joint as little as possible, and support it in the most comfortable position. Put an injured arm or shoulder in a sling (p. 17) or support the leg on a cushion. Watch the circulation in toes and fingers. Get to hospital in sitting position if an arm is injured, in lying position if a leg is injured.

RECOGNIZING A DISLOCATED JOINT

When one or more bones forming a joint are displaced from their normal positions the result is a disclocation. The casualty will have very severe pain and be unable to move the joint. There may be swelling, bruising and some deformity near the joint.

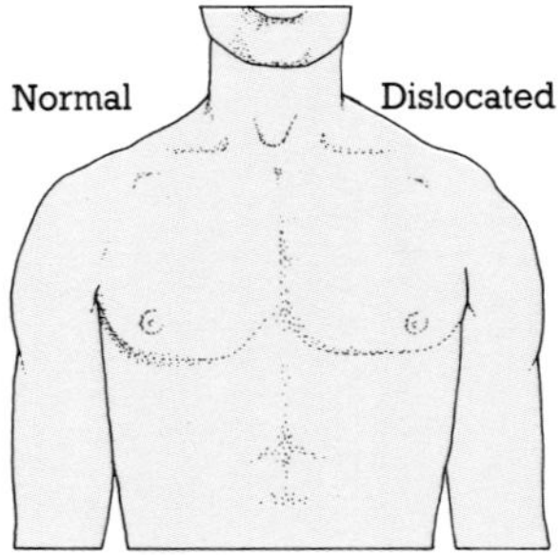

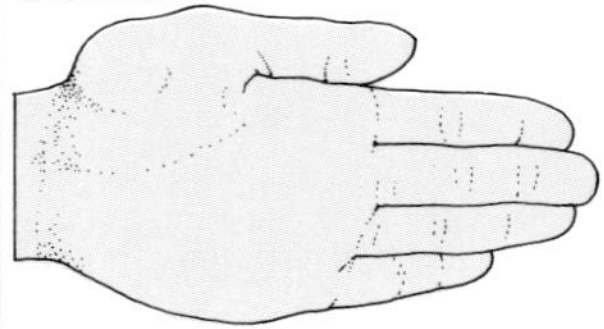

Dislocated joints
There is usually a visible sign of dislocation in the vicinity of the injury. Do not, under any circumstances, attempt to manipulate the joint.

Poisoning

General

Poisons are substances which can harm or kill the body. They can be taken into the body through the mouth, skin or lungs. Even medicines can be poisons if taken in the wrong dose, or by someone for whom they were not prescribed. Poisons commonly found in the home and garden include: Medicines – sleeping tablets, pain-killers, tranquillizers; domestic bleaches, disinfectants, oven cleaners; paraffin, petrol, weed-killers, chemical fertilizers, insecticides, paint and decorating products; food which is decomposing, toadstools and other fungi, green potatoes, berries such as deadly nightshade; rat and mouse poisons; alcohol.

Most cases of poisoning are accidental, and could have been prevented. Children and elderly people are the chief victims.

Treatment of poisoning by mouth

Wash any remaining poison away from the face with water.

If the casualty is unconscious, clear the airway and give artificial

POTENTIAL KILLERS

Many household chemicals, medicines and drugs are lethal if consumed by children – so keep all dangerous substances safely out of their reach.

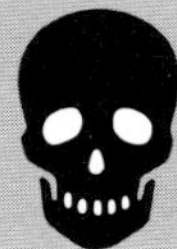

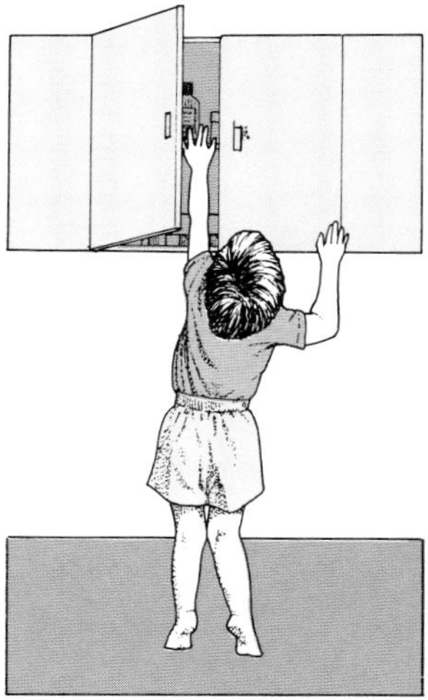

Security

Make sure that cupboards holding drugs, etc., are securely locked.

Poisoning

Treatment *continued*

respiration (p. 13) if necessary. It may be wise, especially if the casualty is suspected of having swallowed a corrosive poison, to give mouth to *nose* resuscitation. In any event, proceed with great care. Check the pulse rate. If breathing regularly, put in the recovery position (p. 13) with head slightly lower than the body (a child could be held over a knee in this position on the way to hospital). Do not leave unattended and watch breathing carefully.
If the casualty is conscious, try to find out what poison was taken, how much, and when. Do not make the casualty vomit, but if he vomits naturally, keep it for identification.
Give nothing by mouth. Watch, in case casualty becomes unconscious.
Get to hospital quickly taking any available evidence of the poison, e.g. an empty bottle or container, sample of plant or berries, tablets or drug. In cases of attempted suicide, there may be no evidence at all of the poison.

TREATMENT OF POISONED BUT CONSCIOUS CASUALTY

- Wash any remaining poison away from casualty's mouth and face.
- Do not give anything by mouth.
- Do not make the casualty vomit.
- Find out what was taken.
- Find out how much.
- Find out when.
- Watch, in case casualty becomes unconscious.
- Get casualty to hospital quickly.

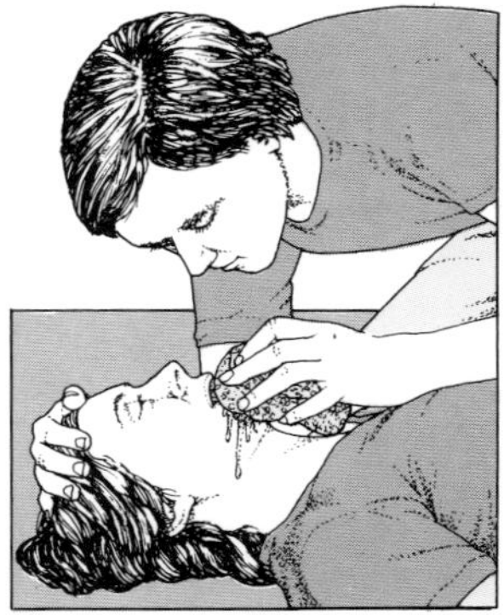

Remove remaining poison
Whether the casualty is conscious or unconscious, wash any remaining poison away from the mouth and face using cold water.

Poisoning

Poisoning through skin	This can be by injection, as in the case of drugs (see *treatment for unconsciousness, p. 43)*, by animal or insect stings or snake bites (see under *Home Treatment, Bites and Stings*). Poisoning is also possible by absorption through the skin. This is particularly so with pesticides.
Signs of poisoning by pesticides	Known contact with pesticide. Casualty may develop convulsions and gradually become unconscious.
Treatment of poisoning by pesticides	If the casualty is unconscious put in the recovery position (p. 13). Keep the airway clear and get to hospital quickly, taking the poison container for identification. If conscious, reassure the casualty and get him to rest. Give as much fluid to drink as possible. Remove contaminated clothing carefully. Get to hospital.
Poisoning into lungs	(See *Gassing*, under *Breathing* p. 36).

IDENTIFYING THE CAUSE OF POISONING
It is important to give the doctor or hospital any information that may be available about the poison the casualty has taken. If the casualty is unconscious, look for an empty drugs bottle or other suspect container but do not waste time looking for possibilities. If the casualty vomits, take a sample to the hospital.

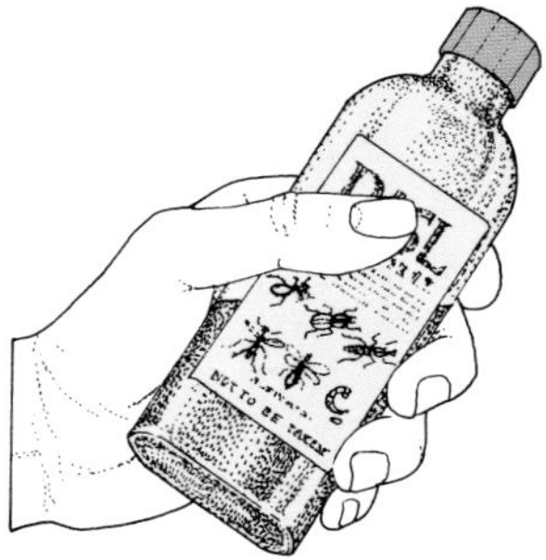

To assist diagnosis
Even if the casualty can tell you what he has taken, a sample of the pill, chemical, berry, fungus – or even an empty container – will still be useful to the doctors.

HOME TREATMENT

Most of the following injuries and ailments are familiar to any household and, in general, can be treated adequately at home. In cases where medical help may be required, this is indicated.

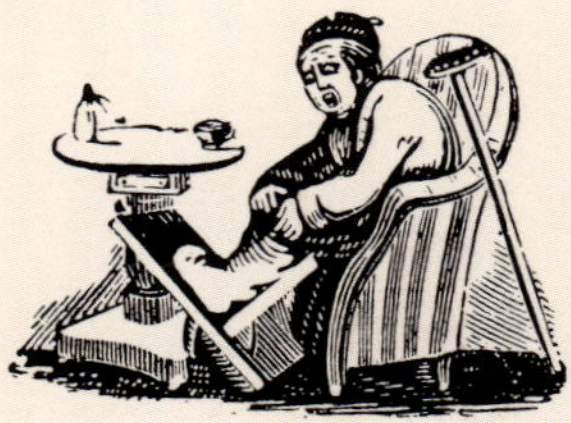

Bites/Stings/Scratches

Animal bites and scratches	Wash thoroughly with water. If bleeding is severe, stop by direct pressure. Cover with a dry, sterile dressing. See a doctor in case an anti-tetanus injection is necessary.
Snake Bites	Snake bites can cause severe pain and the casualty is often very frightened. It is important to identify the snake so that appropriate treatment can be given. In countries where poisonous snakes are common, stocks of anti-venom serum are usually kept in treatment centres.
Treatment for snake bites	Calm the casualty and make him lie down. Clean the wound with water and wash off any venom. Do not cut or suck the bite, or put anything on it. Cover with a dry, sterile dressing. Immobilize the limb and support it. Get the casualty to hospital as soon as possible. If the snake has been killed, take it for identification. If breathing stops, give artificial respiration (p. 13).

ANIMAL BITES
In countries where rabies is present, all bites must be reported and proper medical treatment obtained.

ACTION IN CASE OF SNAKE BITES

- Calm and reassure the casualty
- Flush the wound with water
- Cover with a dry dressing
- Immobilize a bitten limb
- Get casualty to hospital

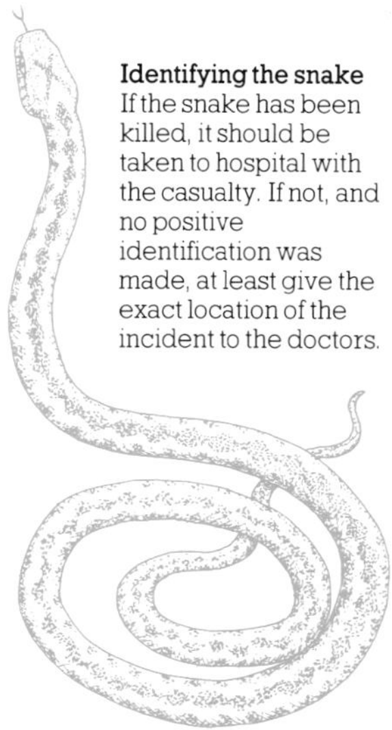

Identifying the snake
If the snake has been killed, it should be taken to hospital with the casualty. If not, and no positive identification was made, at least give the exact location of the incident to the doctors.

Bites/Stings/Scratches

Insect stings (bees, hornets, wasps)

When an insect stings, venom is injected into the skin causing inflammation and local pain. In cases of acute allergies and extra-sensitivity to stings, there may be a severe reaction. even loss of consciousness. If this occurs, put in the recovery position (p. 13). Seek medical aid urgently.

Treatment for stings in the skin

If the sting and poison bag is left in the skin, remove them with tweezers. Put the tweezers on the part of the bag nearest the skin to prevent more poison being squeezed into the skin. A bee sting has a barb on its end, so ease it out gently. Treat as a minor wound and apply dressing.

Treatment for stings in the mouth

Stings in the mouth can cause swelling, leading to difficulty in breathing. Give ice cubes to suck and get the casualty to a doctor. If he becomes unconscious, put in the recovery position (p. 13). If there is no difficulty with breathing, a solution of bicarbonate of soda may help.

INSECT STINGS

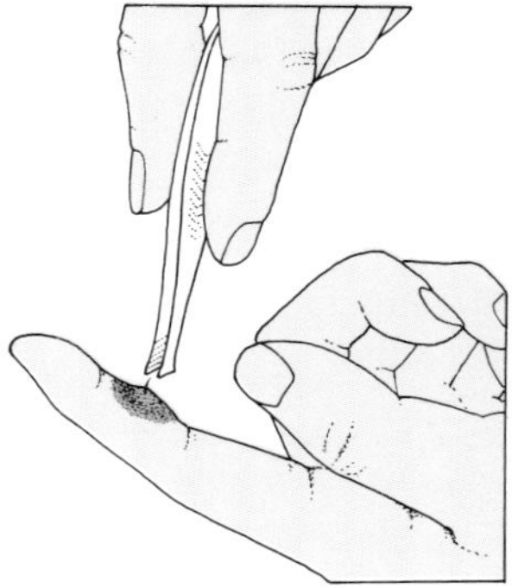

Stings on body or limbs
Remove the sting from the bite with a pair of tweezers, wash the wound and apply a sterile dressing.

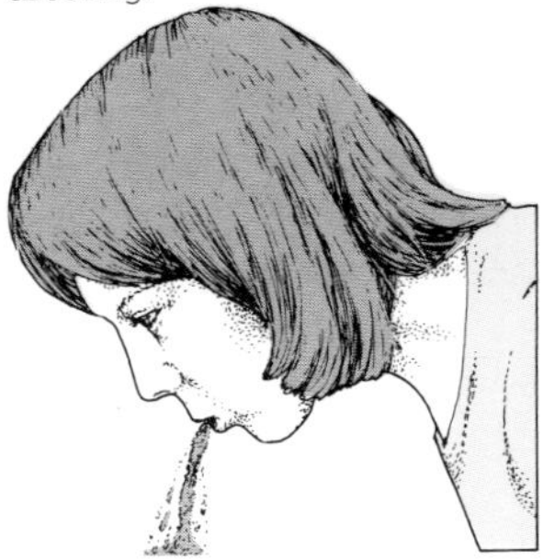

Stings to mouth
Rinsing the mouth with a solution of sodium bicarbonate may be helpful. Sucking ice cubes will help to reduce swelling.

Minor wounds

Minor wounds (cuts, scratches, grazes)	However small a break in the skin, it is a possible entry for germs, so every care must be taken to prevent infection.
Treatment for bleeding	Wash hands well before dressing the wound. Do not touch, or cough, or breathe over the wound. Stop any bleeding by pressure on the dressing over the wound or by fingers near wound. Clean the wound and surrounding skin. If it is as clean as possible and covered with a dry, sterile dressing only, then natural healing will take place by the formation of a dry seal over the wound. Clean the skin thoroughly around the wound with swabs, but do not wipe any dirt towards the wound. Use diluted antiseptic or running water (away from home, 'Antiseptic Wipes' can be used). Wipe away any loose pieces of dirt or debris. Cut away any hairs around the wound. Clean the wound itself – the casualty can often do it under

HYGIENE
Before dressing a wound, wash your hands well – and do not cough or breathe over the wound. Clean the surrounding area, but do not wipe any dirt towards the wound.

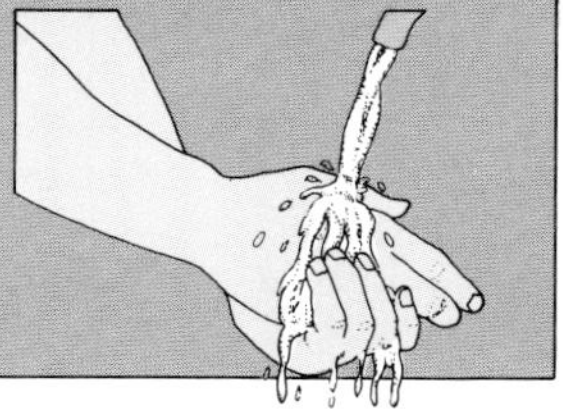

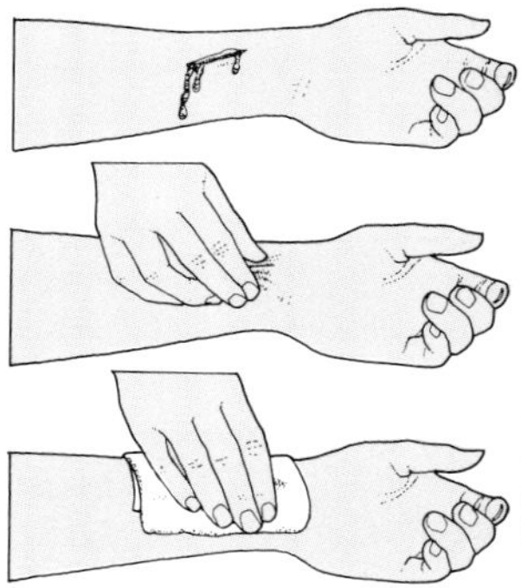

To stop bleeding
Use your fingers to hold the sides of the wound together, or apply pressure through a dressing held over the wound Do not use fluffy material.

Minor wounds

Treatment *continued*	running water – and dry thoroughly. Do not disturb any blood clots because this will re-start bleeding. There is no need to apply ointment or iodine. Cover the wound with a dry, sterile dressing and bandage. If there is a raw area around the wound or a small surface burn, use a non-adhesive dressing, and bandage. Cover small abrasions with adhesive dressings.
Dirty wounds	If there is much dirt in the wound, see a doctor in case an anti-tetanus injection is necessary.
Persistent bleeding	If bleeding persists, despite pressure and dressing, see a doctor.
Deep cuts	If a cut is deep, it may need stitches and protection against infection, so see a doctor.
Removing and changing dressings	Most minor wounds heal within a week. If a dressing has stuck, soak it before removing. Dressings need renewing only if they become wet or soiled.

DRESSING A WOUND

- Clean the wound and the surrounding area.
- Cover the wound with a sterile dressing.
- Firmly bandage the dressing in position.
- Secure the bandage with a safety pin or by slitting and tying.

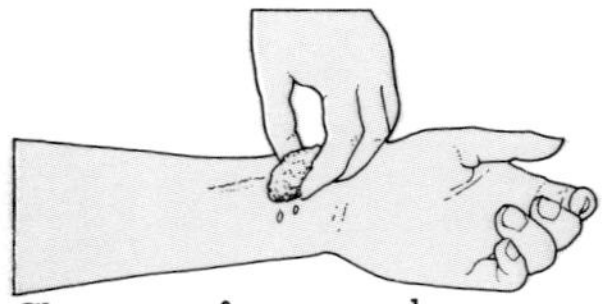

Clean away from wound

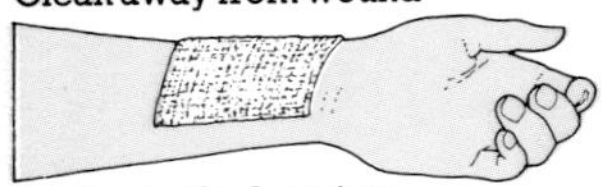

Apply sterile dressing

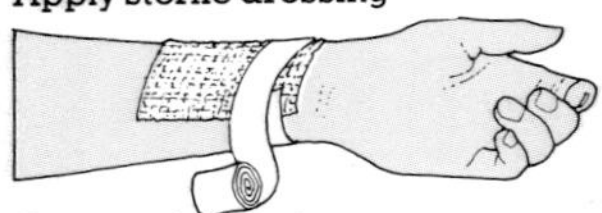

Secure with bandage

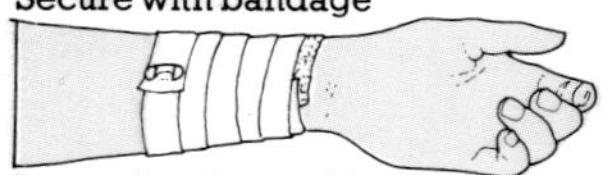

Secure bandage with pin

If bleeding persists and soaks through the dressing, do not remove the original dressing but apply more on top.

Nose bleed

Nose bleeding

This is common in young children and can be caused by a bang on the nose, or by blowing the nose too hard. It can occur suddenly in elderly people suffering from high blood pressure.
Bleeding from the nose after a blow on the head can indicate a fractured skull.

Treatment for nose bleeding

Do not plug the nose. Sit the casualty upright in a chair, preferably near an open window. Tilt the head slightly forward, to prevent blood running back down the throat. Spit out any blood in the mouth and let blood drip from nose into bowl. Tell casualty to pinch the soft part of the nostrils firmly together for 5-10 minutes, and to breathe through his mouth, then release slowly. If bleeding continues, repeat for a further 5 minutes. Do not blow the nose for some hours after bleeding, and keep breathing through mouth to allow blood clot to remain undisturbed. If bleeding persists, or if there are continued bouts of bleeding, see a doctor.

SELF HELP FOR MINOR WOUNDS

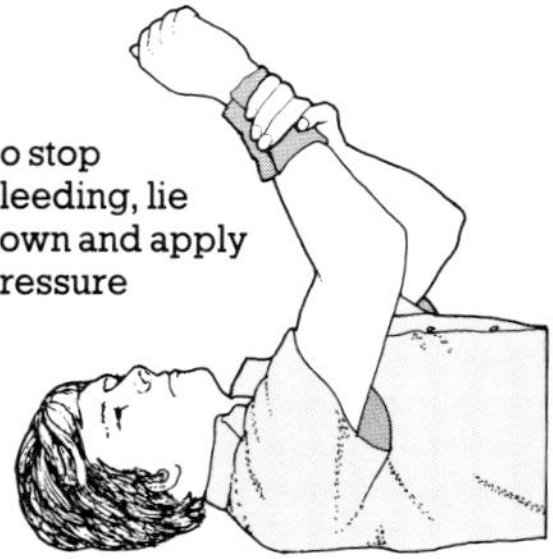

To stop bleeding, lie down and apply pressure

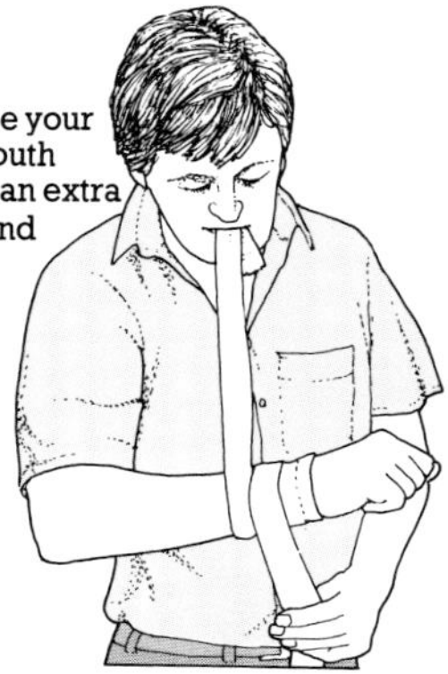

Use your mouth as an extra hand

Self help

On most occasions, you can give yourself the necessary first aid for minor wounds. If you have cut an arm or hand, it is a good idea to lie down, raise the limb and apply pressure to the wound. Use your teeth to help with bandaging.

Ear bleed/Bruise

Ear, bleeding from	Control bleeding from the outer part of the ear by direct pressure on the cut and treat as a cut. Bleeding from the inner ear is more serious and will require attention from a doctor. Get casualty to lie down and cover the whole ear with a pad or dressing, and bandage round the head. Keep the head inclined down on the side of the injury. If unconscious, put in the recovery position (p. 13), with head slightly lower, still keeping the affected ear downwards. Get to hospital.
Bruise	A bruise is bleeding from tiny blood vessels under the skin following injury. There is usually discolouration and pain.
Treatment for bruises	Check for further injuries, because bruising can accompany a fracture. Rest the affected part to allow the blood to clot. Raise an injured limb. Apply a cold compress or ice pack to help reduce pain. Minor bruises heal without further treatment.

NOSE BLEED

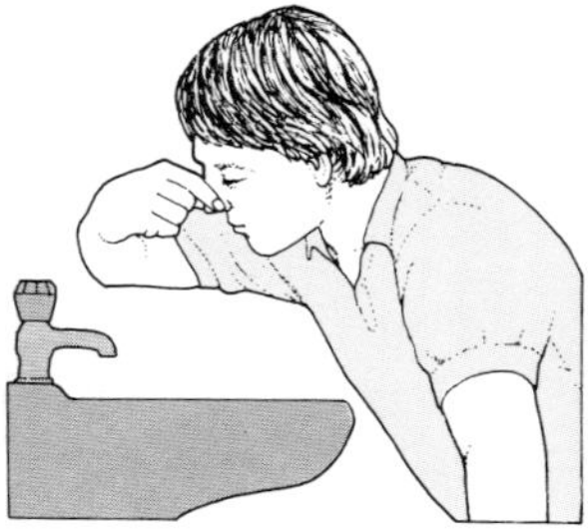

Treatment
Lean over a bowl or basin, and pinch the soft part of the nose while breathing through your mouth.

EAR BLEEDING
If the source of bleeding is not apparent, there may be an internal injury. Get the casualty to hospital quickly.

●
How to make a cold compress
Soak some absorbent material, e.g. a towel, handkerchief or cotton wool, in cold water. Squeeze out the cloth and apply it to the bruise or injury.

●
How to make an ice pack
Fill a plastic bag with ice, preferably crushed, and add some salt which will improve the cooling effects. Tie the bag and wrap it in a towel.

Minor burns & scalds

Burns and scalds, minor

The only type of burns and scalds which should receive home treatment alone are those involving small areas of skin, i.e. not larger than about 2.5 cm (1 inch) square.
If burns affect eyelids or the face, always see a doctor.

Treatment for burns and scalds

As with severe burns, immediate treatment must be to cool the burned tissue to prevent further damage and to relieve pain. Either immerse in cold water, or put under a running cold tap, until pain has eased. Treat the burned area as a wound. Clean around it, carefully pat it dry and then apply a dry or non-adhesive dressing only, and bandage in place.

Friction burns

Friction burns can be caused by running a rope through one's hands, as in climbing or sailing. They can be very painful.

Treatment for friction burns

Immerse burned area in cold water. When the pain has lessened, dry gently and cover with dressing.

THE SKIN

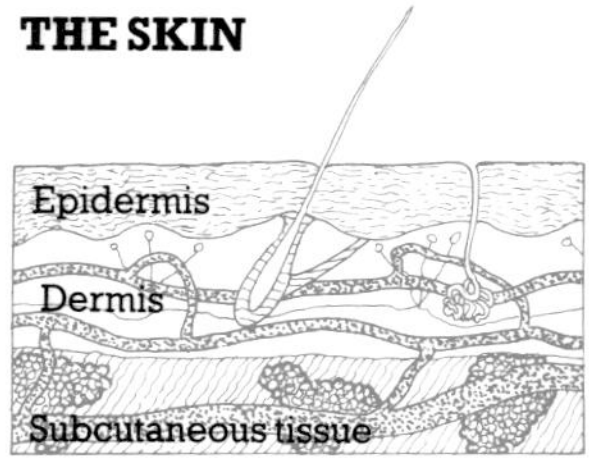

What does the skin do?
The skin is a vital protective layer which form the outer covering of the body. Its functions include the regulation of heat: restricting heat loss in cold conditions through a reduced blood supply to the surface; losing heat in hot conditions by increasing the blood supply and by evaporation (sweating). The skin is also responsible for retention of body fluids and, through the nerve endings contained in the dermis, warning the brain of danger.

TYPES OF BURN

Superficial
In superficial burns, only the outer layer of skin, the epidermis, is destroyed. These burns are very painful but generally heal well. The problem is one of fluid loss if the burn is extensive.

Deep
In deep burns, the epidermis and the dermis are destroyed. There may be very little pain but these burns heal slowly and leave scars.

Eye injuries

Eye injuries general	All eye injuries can be serious, involving a risk of infection and possible loss of sight. Medical aid should be sought.
Black eye	This is a bruise around the eye, due to bleeding under the skin. The skin becomes discoloured and swelling can develop after injury.
Treatment for black eye	Apply cold compresses or ice packs immediately after injury to help prevent swelling. A black eye can indicate damage to the eye or skull, so see a doctor.
Chemical burn on eye	This is a serious injury, requiring immediate treatment. First aid is given on page 56.
Eye wound	This can be caused by a blow, a scratch from an animal or flying objects.
Treatment for eye wound	Get the casualty to lie down. Close the eyelid, cover with a dressing and bandage. Get to hospital.

REMOVING FOREIGN BODY FROM EYE

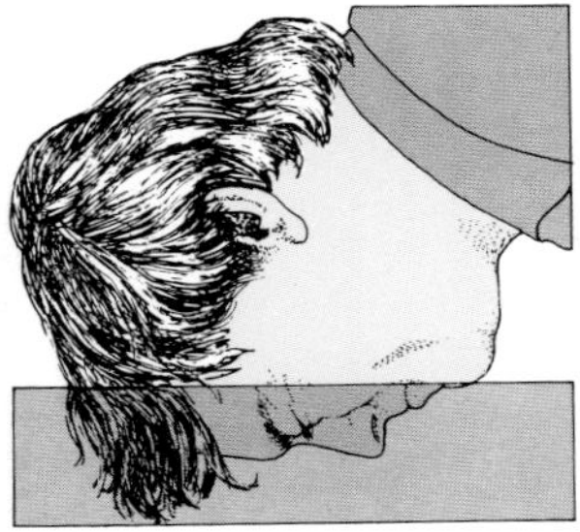

Self help
Objects can be dislodged from the eye by immersion in water, or by gently drawing the eyelid over the eye while looking down.

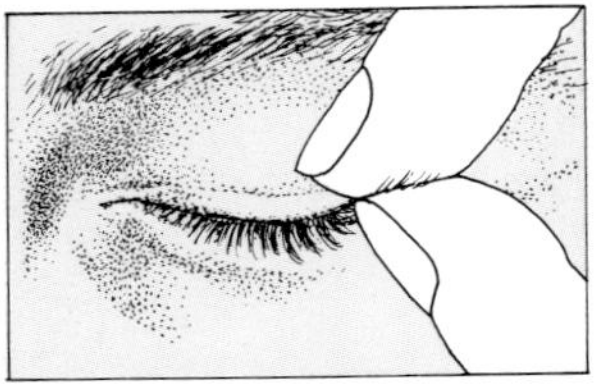

IF OBJECT IS EMBEDDED OR EYE IS WOUNDED
Do not attempt to remove the object or agitate the eye. Get the casualty to lie down, cover the eye with a dressing and bandage to restrict movement. Take the casualty to hospital.

Fits/Fainting

Convulsions and fits (in young children)	These are not related to Epilepsy (p. 45) and usually occur in young children who are suffering from raised temperatures and infection.
Signs of convulsions and fits	The child becomes stiff and arches his back and holds his breath; his limbs may twitch, and there can be frothing at the mouth. His face becomes red or blue and his eyes roll up.
Treatment for convulsions	Loosen tight clothing. A small baby can be wrapped in a sheet or blanket. Put in the recovery position (p. 13) if possible and cover with one blanket. If the body temperature is high, sponge with tepid water, and wipe froth from mouth. Send for a doctor.
Fainting	Fainting is a short period of unconsciousness (see p. 43) following a decrease in the amount of blood reaching the brain. Those most likely to be affected are children, young adults, elderly persons. Causes

SIGNS OF CONVULSIONS

- Stiffness of body
- Arching of back
- Twitching of limbs
- Frothing at mouth
- Face turns red or blue
- Eyes roll upwards

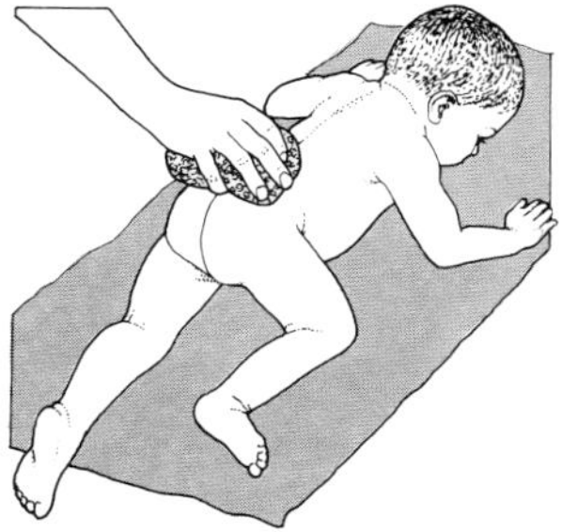

Reduce body heat
If the body temperature is high, sponge with tepid water and wipe froth from mouth.

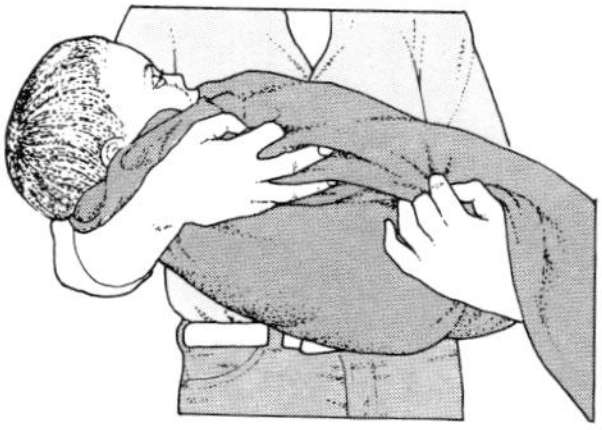

Handling casualty
Babies can be better handled if they are wrapped in a sheet or a blanket.

Fits/Fainting

	include: lack of air, hunger, tiredness, heat, standing in one position for a long time, fright, injury.
Signs of fainting	Casualty feels unsteady, giddy and may start to sweat and feel sick. Pulse is weak and slow at first but will increase in speed; unconsciousness follows.
Treatment for fainting	If there is no danger from fire, traffic, etc. place in the recovery position (p. 13), in fresh air if possible. Place the head slightly lower than the body. Loosen tight clothing at neck, chest and waist. The casualty should recover consciousness within few minutes. When conscious, give sips of water; later, a drink such as tea may be helpful. After rest, recovery should be complete. If not, the casualty should be taken to hospital. If a person is feeling faint but is in a place where it is not possible to lie down, such as a crowded hall – he should put his head between his knees.

FAINTING

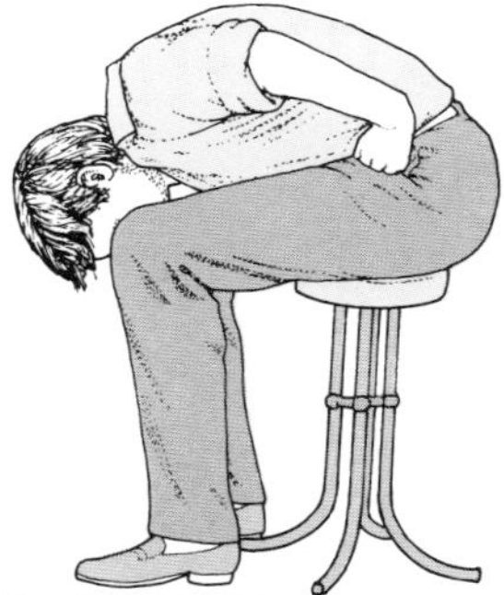

When feeling faint
A person who feels faint in a place where it is impossible to lie down should place his head between his knees.

ASTHMA ATTACKS

An asthma attack can be quite alarming, especially if it is accompanied by acute shortage of breath and restriction of the breathing passages. Known sufferers are often able to deal with an attack by themselves. If not, or if an attack has not been experienced before, the casualty should be put into a comfortable, relaxed position (not lying down) and given plenty of fresh air. Asthma is sometimes caused by an allergy – to dust or animal fur for example – so fresh air will help to reduce the effects of such irritants.

Foreign bodies

Description	A foreign body is anything which should not be in the body or in a wound, or an object which is swallowed, inhaled or is lodged in an eye, nose or ear. It can include dirt (in a wound), pieces of glass, metal, small coins, beads, safety-pins etc.
General treatment for foreign bodies	Remove only loose foreign bodies. Leave those which do not lift out easily; do not prise or force them. If applying a bandage, do not put pressure on the wound. Any large hooks, such as fish-hooks, caught in the skin should be seen and removed by a doctor. An anti-tetanus injection may be required.
Foreign body in eye	See under *"Eye Injuries" p. 77.*
Inhaled foreign body	If choking occurs, *see p. 34.* If not, and the foreign body remains in the nose or throat, take the casualty to a doctor. In unusual cases it may be necessary to force air past the obstruction.

MAKING A RING PAD
If a foreign body is embedded in a wound, do not attempt to remove it unless it comes away easily. Dress the wound with a ring pad to avoid direct pressure.

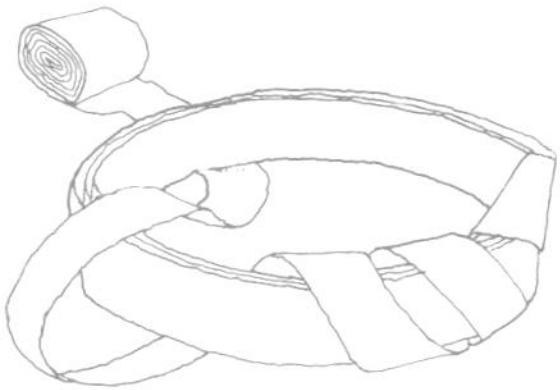

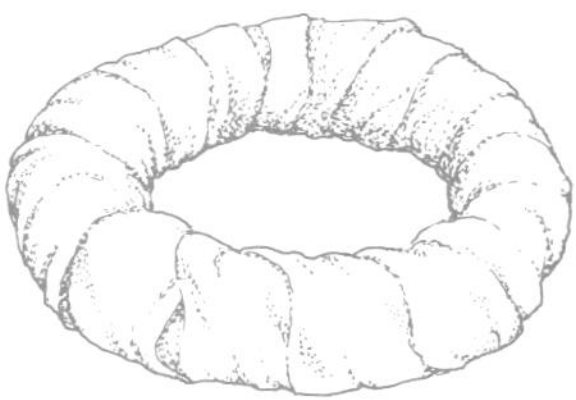

Ring pad
Make a loop with two or three turns of a narrow bandage. Take the free end and wind it firmly around the loop until a neat ring is formed. Place the pad around the wound and bandage.

Foreign bodies

Foreign body in wound	See *Bleeding, p. 39.*
Foreign body in nose or ear	Young children tend to put objects such as peas or beads in the nose or ear. Unless it is actually sticking out, do not attempt to remove it, and do not pour anything into the ear.
Treatment for foreign bodies in nose or ear	Tell the casualty to breath through the mouth (if the nose is affected), and take him to hospital. If the casualty is a child with the object lodged in an ear, prevent him from poking it by covering the ear with a bandage.
Swallowed foreign bodies	This usually occurs when a small object suddenly slips to the back of the throat and cannot be brought foward by the tongue.
Treatment for swallowed foreign bodies	If choking occurs, *see page 34.* If the object swallowed is sharp, such as a piece of glass, a fish bone or an open safety-pin, give nothing by mouth and get the casualty to a doctor at once.

DRESSING A WOUND WITH A FOREIGN BODY IN IT

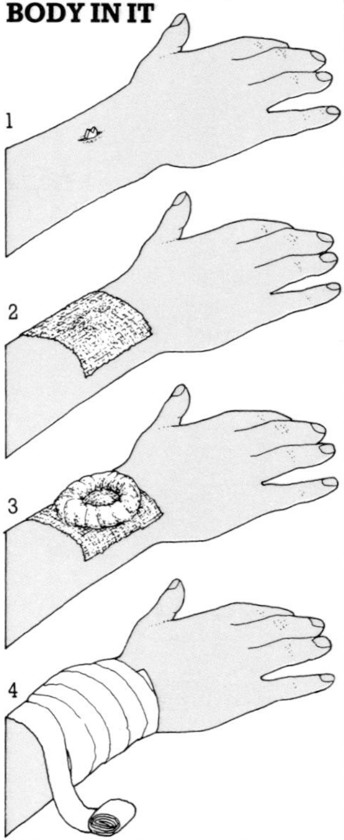

1 Make sure the surrounding area is clean.
2 Place a dry gauze dressing over the wound.
3 Put ring pad over gauze.
4 Bandage over dressing.

Muscular injuries

Cramp	Cramp is a sudden pain and tightness in the muscles – the leg muscles being most often affected.
Treatment for cramp	Stretch the affected muscle, e.g. if cramp is in the calf of the leg, straighten the knee and pull the foot up towards the shin. This will force the opposite set of muscles to contract, so that the affected muscles will relax, and the pain disappear.
Sprain	A sprain occurs at a joint after wrenching and tearing of the ligaments.
Signs of sprain	Pain, especially on movement; swelling and bruising later.
Treatment for sprain	Put the casualty in a comfortable position. Uncover the joint, then pad and bandage firmly to give support. If an ankle is injured, the bandage can be put over a shoe. If an arm, put it in a sling. Sprained joints should be x-rayed in case of fracture.

SWALLOWED FOREIGN BODIES

Usually all that is required to dislodge an object from the throat is to tilt the body until the object is naturally ejected by coughing. With a heavily built adult, this may not be so easy. It is important, therefore, not to panic. If the object is sharp, and has been swallowed completely, the casualty should see a doctor.

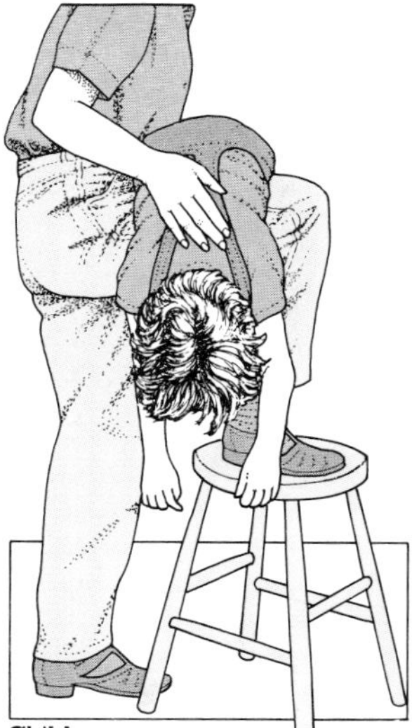

Children
A child with an object lodged in the throat can be placed over an adult's knee and slapped three or four times on the back.

Muscular injuries

Strain	A strain occurs when a muscle has been pulled or over-stretched so that the muscle fibres have been torn. It can follow sudden severe exertion or the lifting of heavy weights.
Signs of strain	Sudden pain, which is worse on movement. Sometimes bruising and swelling. Onset of cramp.
Treatment of strain	Put casualty in a comfortable position and support the injured part until it can be seen by a doctor.
'Stitch'	A pain in the side of the abdomen, occurring during games and running. No treatment is necessary, just stop and rest.
Winding	Winding is caused by a blow in the upper abdomen, which may cause the casualty to double up with pain.
Treatment of winding	Let casualty stay in the most comfortable position until the pain passes. If there is loss of consciousness, put in the recovery position (p. 13).

CRAMP

A tightening and loss of elasticity in a muscle is called cramp. It is painful to a variable degree and may, during exercise, preceed muscular strain (pulled muscle). Sometimes, during running, cramp can be confused with a pulled muscle – so it is advisable to stop until the pain passes off or injury is confirmed. Cramp is sometimes caused by a lack of salt, especially in hot weather. Salt tablets, or a weak solution of salt in water should help considerably. Games players and athletes should ensure that their diet contains sufficient salt.

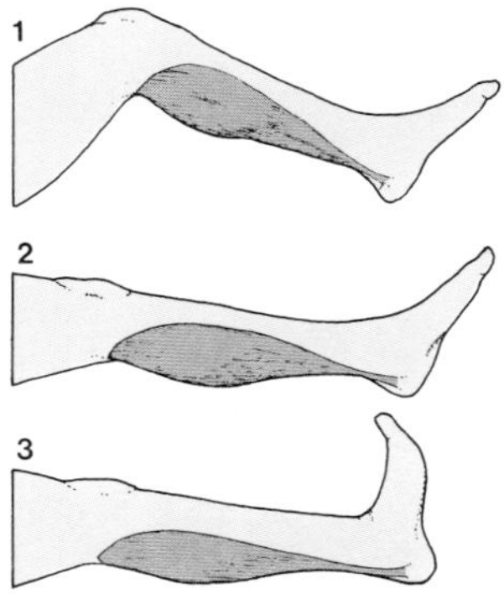

Cramp in calf
Cramp in the calf muscle can be relieved by straightening the leg and gently pulling back the foot.

SAFETY & SURVIVAL

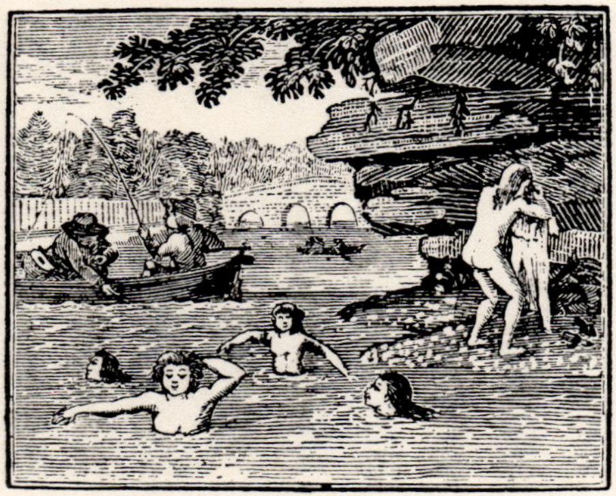

Safety

Although accidents are bound to happen, most can be prevented by commonsense precautions. Casualty figures indicate that it is the very young and the elderly who are most in danger.

Infants

Children up to the age of 5 years are accident-prone because they do not see danger. They can be victims of falls, poisoning, burns, choking, suffocation, cuts – many caused by adult carelessness in the home. Small children need protection against strong sunshine, which can cause extensive loss of body fluid through sweating, and protected in very low temperatures against a fall in their body heat.

Older children

Older children may be aware of danger but are more adventurous so that they may incur injuries during games, in water sports and on the roads.

Adults

Adults may see possible dangers, but still cause accidents through lack of thought and sheer carelessness. Injuries occur at work, in sport, on the roads, and in the home and garden.

Elderly people

Elderly people need to become more accident-conscious as they grow older. As the body gradually slows down, it takes longer to carry out any preventive action, such as avoiding a fall. Watch out for hazards in the home; see that there is good lighting and handrails, wear shoes rather than slippers for better support and balance.

Old people who live alone are prone to dangers, especially if they continue to clean windows and climb on chairs to reach shelves – just as they have always done. A fall and broken bone may not be serious for a young child or a healthy adult, but in an elderly person with more brittle bones, it can lead to permanent disablement.

Falls are the most common cause of death from accidents in the home. Elderly people, especially women, are most at risk. Burns and scalds occur through carelessness with unguarded fires, cigarettes and when cooking. Poisoning can result from taking the wrong tablets absentmindedly.

Being safety-conscious must lead to fewer unnecessary accidents, and prevent much injury and suffering.

CARRYING INJURED CASUALTIES

It is sometimes necessary to move a casualty – usually when there is danger in not doing so. Below are some methods for carrying casualties effectively.

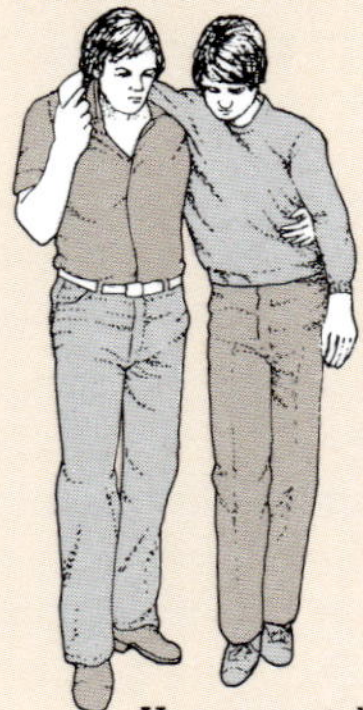

Human crutch

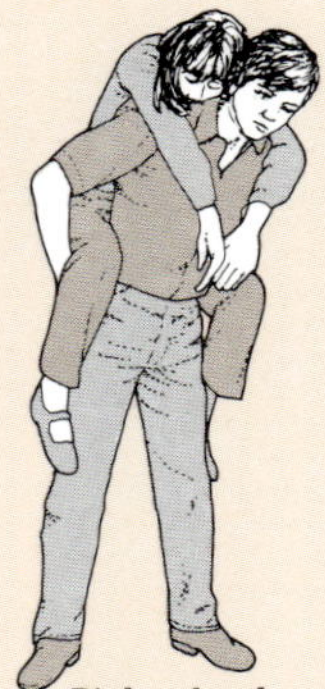

Pick-a-back

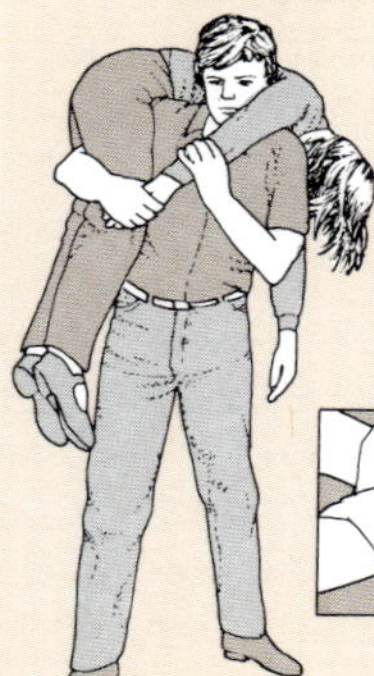

Fireman's lift

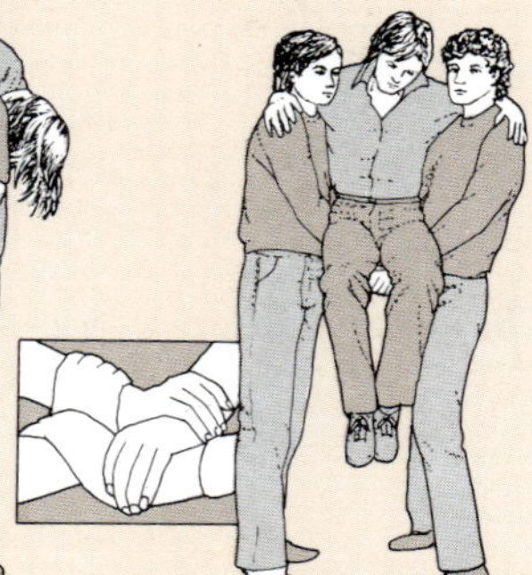

Four handed seat

Survival

Exposure to extreme heat and cold	Excess of heat or cold can cause serious damage to the body, even death, so it is worth being well prepared in order that the body can adjust to the outside air temperature.
Effects of heat	The body temperature, normally about 37°C (98.4°F) is kept constant by the cooling effect of evaporation of moisture from the skin, or sweating. When the outside temperature is high, we sweat more, and more water and salt is lost from the body and this affects the blood circulation.
Avoiding heat disorders	Gradually get used to heat before being energetic, and wear loose, light clothes. Protect the head from hot sun and drink plenty of cool fluids, take more salt at meals.
Heat exhaustion	Heat exhaustion occurs when sweating is excessive, so there is abnormal loss of salt and water from the body under hot and humid conditions. The onset can be slow and can affect the physically fit.

HEAT DISORDERS
To avoid heat disorders: wear loose, light clothing. Protect the head and the neck from direct sun. Avoid strenuous exercise. Drink plenty of cool drinks. Take extra salt.

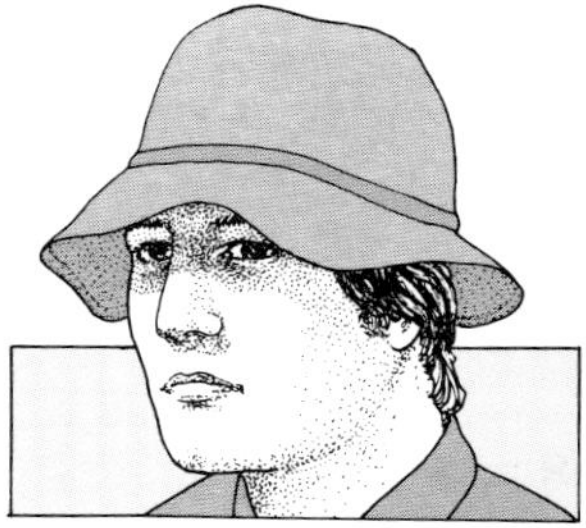
Wear protective clothing

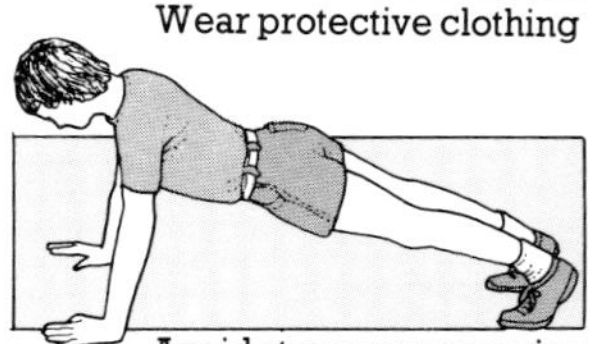
Avoid strenuous exercise

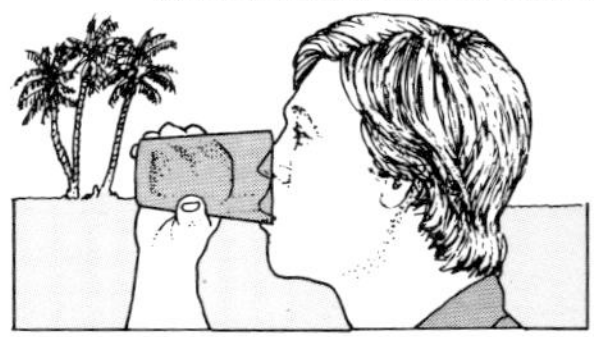
Drink plenty of cool fluids, and take extra salt.

Causes of heat exhaustion	Strenuous exercise in heat; inadequate precautions by newcomers to hot climates
Signs of heat exhaustion	Physical and mental exhaustion; onset of cramp; pale, clammy skin; slow, weak pulse. The body temperature will be near normal.
Treatment of heat exhaustion	Keep in cool, shady surrounding and give drinks of half tsp. (5ml) salt to 0.6 litre (1 pint) of water. See a doctor if there is no improvement.
Heat stroke	Heat stroke can come on suddenly, and is serious because the heat-regulating system of the body breaks down so that the body cannot control its temperature by sweating.
Signs of heat stroke	The body temperature will be very high. The skin will be flushed, but will feel dry and burning. The victim will probably have a headache and a fast, strong pulse. His mental condition may be confused and this can lead to unconsciousness.

TREATMENT FOR HEAT DISORDERS

It is essential, in all cases to move the casualty into the shade before treatment.

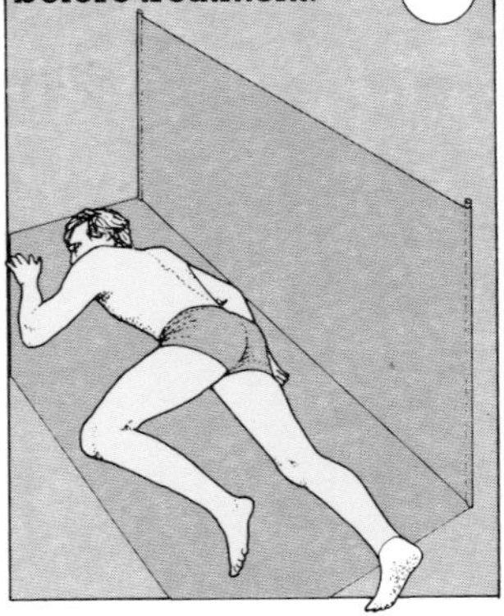

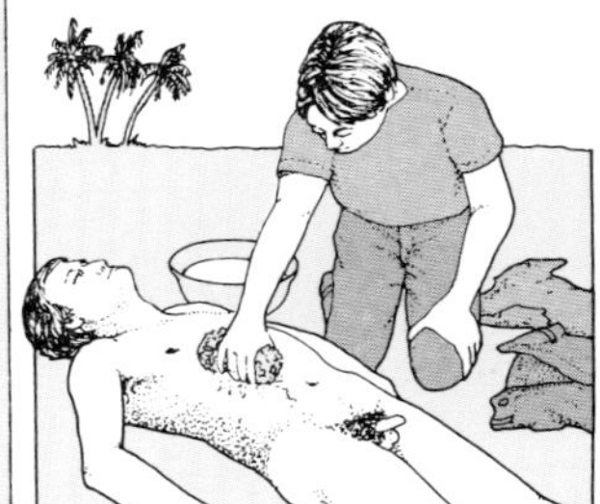

Treatment
Remove the casualty's clothing and sponge the body with tepid (not cold) water.

Survival

Treatment of heatstroke

It is essential to cool the body and reduce the temperature. Put the casualty in the shade, remove clothing and sponge the body with tepid (not cold) water. Apply a cold compress to the forehead. If the casualty is unconscious, put in the recovery position (p. 13) and let direct currents of air fan the body.

When the casualty is conscious keep him cool. See a doctor.

Sunburn

Sunburn is a burned condition of the skin due to over-exposure to the sun's rays. Fair-skinned persons and young children are especially prone to sunburn and need adequate protection. It can also occur in conditions of ice, snow or desert sand, where the ultra-violet rays (which are responsible for browning the skin) are reflected from these surfaces.

Treatment of sunburn

Keep in the shade and keep cool. Calamine cream will soothe reddened skin. If severely affected, treat for Burns (p. 54).

SUNBURN

Remember that burning by the sun can produce the same effects as other kinds of burning. The treatment, therefore, should be as for burns. In mild cases, calamine lotion can be used to soothe reddened skin. For serious cases *see page 53.*

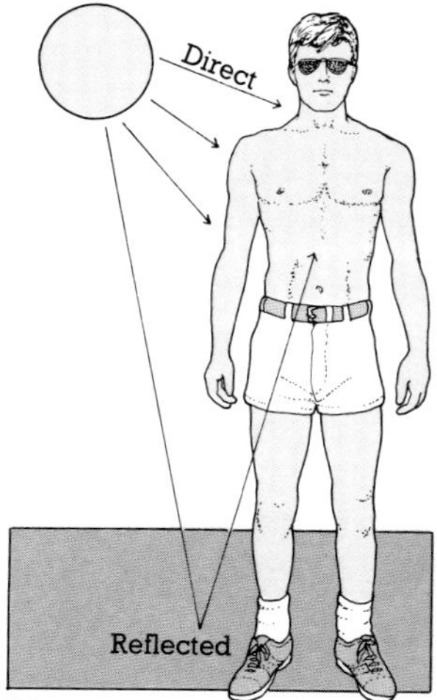

Direct and reflected sunburn
Burns may be received not only from direct sunlight but also when reflected by water, sand, snow etc.

Survival

Effects of cold

This is not just a hazard in snow and ice, but in all outdoor activities and water sports, where there is danger of exposure to cold and wet conditions. Such exposure, often accompanied by physical tiredness, will cause a drop in body temperature and can lead to collapse due to exposure.

Prevention of exposure

Dress warmly and adequately, and have added light-weight, waterproof protection. Carry reserve dry clothing, such as socks, head-covering and gloves. Do not go walking or climbing in severe terrain or extreme weather conditions unless you are physically fit. Do not carry excess loads. Never go without a trained guide or leader.

Signs of collapse

Slowing down of physical and mental activity; shivering and weakness; irritability; difficulty in speech and sight.
If untreated, there may be collapse, unconsciousness and, possibly, death.

DIET
In countries where extremes of climate may be encountered it is important to eat and drink regularly. In hot climates, take plenty of salt with meals. Salt retains moisture and will help to keep the body's fluids at the right level. Take plenty of cool drinks and avoid periods of prolonged physical exertion.

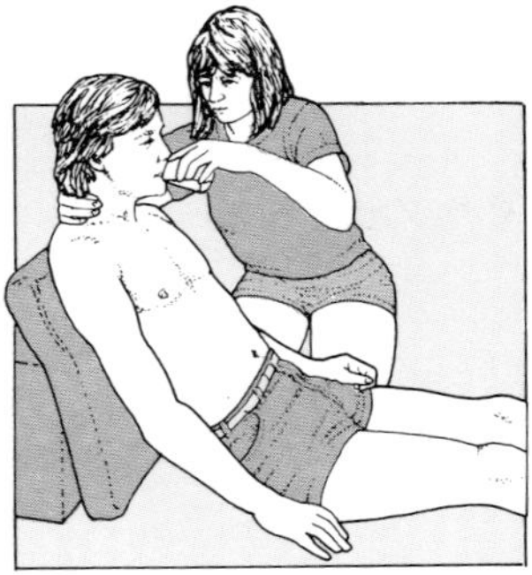

Heat stoke
This is a more serious condition than heat exhaustion. The casualty may have a very high body temperature and a fast, strong pulse. He may be confused and could become unconscious. Reduction of the body temperature is essential. Put the casualty in the shade, remove clothing, sponge with tepid water and administer cold drinks.

Survival

Treatment of collapse through cold

Recognize the signs of collapse and act at once. Immediate treatment is to rest the casualty, and provide shelter and warmth so that there is no further heat loss to the body. Use sleeping bags if they are near at hand, or wrap the casualty in polythene to encourage heat retention. When the rescue party arrives, get the casualty to base on a stretcher. See a doctor on arrival.

Hypothermia

This is a dangerous condition of heat loss from the body, with a consequent dropping of the body temperature.
If no protection against further heat loss is taken, unconsciousness and death will follow.

Causes of hypothermia

Exposure to cold, which can occur at home if there is insufficient room heating, clothing or food. Outside, extreme wintry conditions can be responsible. Those most at risk are babies, elderly people, the physically handicapped.

WIND CHILL FACTOR

The wind can produce the effects of much lower temperatures than those recorded. These tables show how much.

No danger if adequately clothed

Danger of freezing if skin exposed

TEMPERATURE FAHRENHEIT	WIND SPEED MPH						
	5	10	15	20	25	30	35
50	48	40	36	32	30	28	27
40	37	28	22	18	16	13	11
30	27	16	9	4	0	-2	-4
20	16	4	-5	-10	-15	-18	-20
10	6	-9	-18	-25	-29	-33	-35
0	-3	-21	-36	-39	-44	-48	-52
-10	-15	-33	-45	-53	-59	-63	-67
-20	-26	-46	-58	-67	-74	-79	-82
-30	-36	-58	-72	-82	-88	-94	-98

TEMPERATURE CENTIGRADE	WIND SPEED KPH						
	8	16	24	32	40	48	56
10	9	4	2	0	-1	-2	-3
4	3	-2	-5	-8	-9	-10	-12
-1	-3	-9	-13	-15	-18	-19	-20
-7	-9	-15	-20	-23	-26	-28	-29
-12	-14	-23	-28	-32	-34	-36	-37
-18	-19	-29	-38	-39	-42	-44	-49
-23	-26	-36	-43	-47	-50	-53	-55
-29	-32	-43	-50	-55	-59	-62	-63
-34	-38	-50	-58	-63	-67	-70	-72

Survival

Signs of hypothermia	**Babies:** refusal of food, body is very cold, although the skin may have good colour. Child may be very quiet. **Adults:** slow, weak pulse. Casualty is cold and pale, with slow mental and physical reaction.
Treatment of hypothermia	Allow the body temperature to rise gradually by putting casualty between blankets. **Do not use hot-water bottles or electric blankets.** If the casualty is conscious, give warm, sweet drinks. Get to hospital quickly.
Frostbite	This usually occurs where part of the body is exposed to extreme cold. The extremities of the body – ears, nose, fingers and toes are the most commonly affected.
Treatment of frostbite	Put the casualty in a sheltered position and remove any tight clothing from near the frostbitten area. Place affected hands or feet inside a blanket, sleeping bag or clothing. Do not apply direct heat. Get to hospital quickly.

BE PREPARED
To prevent cold exhaustion:
- Dress adequately and warmly
- Have waterproof protection
- Have reserve dry clothing

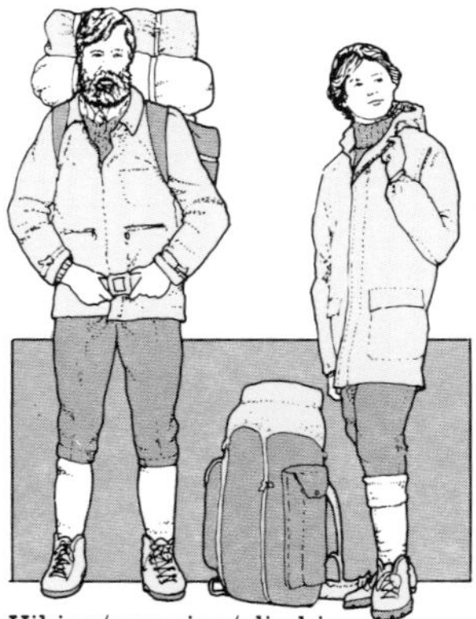

Hiking/camping/climbing
Those who take part in these outdoor activities are the most prone to the effects of cold, but adequate forethought and preparation will eliminate many risks.

HYPOTHERMIA
If a casualty is suffering from hypothermia, it is essential to warm them slowly. Rapid increase of temperature can be fatal.

EMERGENCY SERVICES

NAME/SERVICE	PHONE NUMBER	ADDRESS

Use these pages to record details of essential services: ambulance, doctor, dentist, etc.

NAME/SERVICE	PHONE NUMBER	ADDRESS

INDEX OF EMERGENCY ACTION

Index

Figures in italics refer to illustrations

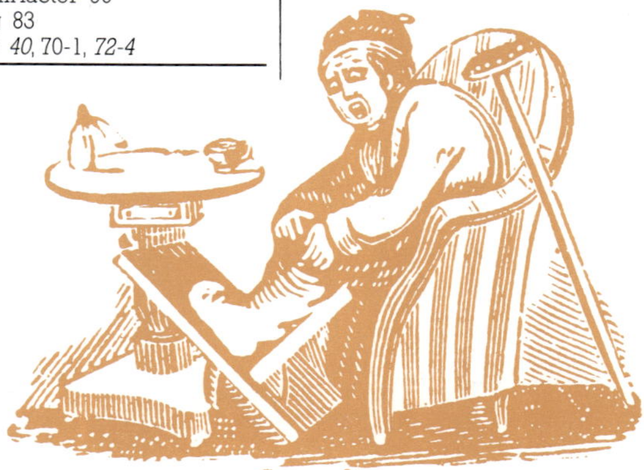

Acknowledgments

The 'How To' Book of First Aid
and Safety was created by
Simon Jennings and Company Limited.
We are grateful to the following
individuals and organisations
for their assistance in the
making of this book:

Hazel Breeden: *picture research*
Nigel Chamberlain: *all line and tone illustrations*
Quentin Courtney: *additional artwork*
John Couzins: *cover and title page photographs*
The Dover Archive: *engravings and embellishments*
Ann Hall: *compilation of index*
Coral Mula: *colour illustrations pages 6, 7, 10, 11, 18*
Catherine Stretton SRN, RCNT, NDN, FETC: *text consultant*
Michael Woods: *colour illustrations pages 22/3, 26/7*

Photographs
John Couzins: pages **14, 15, 31**
Volvo (GB) Limited: page **19** *bl* and *br*
Spectrum Picture Library: pages **19** *t*, **30** *t*, and *b*

abbreviations: *t* top; *b* bottom; *bl* bottom left; *br* bottom right

Typesetting by Text Filmsetters Ltd., Orpington, Kent
Headline setting by Diagraphic Typesetting Ltd., London
Additional display setting by Facet Photosetting, London

Special thanks to Norman Ruffell and
the staff of Swaingrove Ltd., Bury St. Edmunds,
Suffolk, for the lithographic reproduction.